Welcome to the Wealthy Fit Pro Series

The fitness industry is beautifully flawed. It simultaneously transforms lives and chews up and spits out many of its top change agents. If you want to stick around, you must learn what the certification programs *don't* teach: the business and marketing necessary for success.

The *Wealthy Fit Pro Guides* gather the brightest minds in the global fitness industry to bring you the guidance you need at the lowest price possible. You hold in your hands book two in this series: *Online Training*. For many trainers who cut their teeth on in-person training, usually in a gym, starting an online business as a part- or full-time gig can be a gateway to helping more people, making more money, and having more freedom. This book can show you the way.

I embraced the challenge of this series because when I started my career I felt alone. I was lucky to come across mentors and read the right books at the right time. If we want to make the world a better, healthier place, it starts with passionate fit pros like you. You have the potential to change lives, but it won't happen if you can't make the money that you deserve.

I'm happy you're here and excited for your career. Welcome, and let's dig in!

—Coach Jon

*P.S. This book is the beginning. I'd love to connect with you more. Feel free to friend me on my personal Facebook page at **theptdc.com/fb** and send me a message anytime. My entire team and I are here for you.*

Also by Jonathan Goodman and the Personal Trainer
Development Center

Books

The Wealthy Fit Pro's Guides
Starting Your Career (Book 1)
Online Training (Book 2)

*Ignite the Fire: The Secrets to Building a Successful Personal Training
Career* (Revised, Updated, and Expanded)

*Personal Trainer Pocket Book: A Handy Reference for All Your Daily
Questions*

Viralnomics: How to Get People to <u>Want</u> to Talk About You

The Highly Wealthy Online Trainer box set:
Habits of Highly Wealthy Online Trainers (Book 1)
Marketing Breakthroughs of Highly Wealthy Online Trainers (Book 2)

All titles and an updated book list available at
theptdc.com/store.

Children's Book

Adventure, Adventure Awaits For Us All
with Alison Goodman.
Available on Amazon.

Courses & Certifications

Online Trainer Academy
A comprehensive certification in online training.
theptdc.com/ota

Starting Your Career CEC companion course
theptdc.com/syc-cec

Advanced Marketing Resource

Fitness Marketing Monthly — The Complete Collection
theptdc.com/fmm

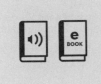

The Wealthy Fit Pro's Guide to Online Training

ISBN: 9781073501946

Cover and interior book design by Growler Media

Bulk order discounts are available for fitness centers, education companies, academic institutions, and mentorships. Please inquire by emailing support@theptdc.com with subject line "bulk book order."

The Wealthy Fit Pro's Guide to

ONLINE TRAINING

—

JONATHAN GOODMAN
AND
ALEX CARTMILL

CONTENTS

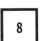
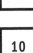

Online Training Is Your Next Step

The fitness industry is designed to abuse trainers.

You're told to follow industry "norms," be a good foot soldier, stick to the rules. Well, I've got some news for you: Industry norms generate average results. They tend to bring everybody to the middle. The middle is safe. And static, since your career never progresses. The business model breaks us down, exhausts us, and leaves us without much money at the end of it all. That's what you get following industry norms.

You have to challenge the norms. You have to listen to and learn from others who have challenged the norms themselves and found a better way. The fit pros who refuse to challenge the status quo become frustrated, burned out, and part of the sorry majority who will have the casket closed at the end of the day wondering where all their time went. Sorry to be so grim, but that's a fact.

No career is automated. You aren't guaranteed to hit certain milestones or achieve levels of skill and income just by showing up. You have to push for what you want. You may just have to go against the grain, too. You know, challenge some norms.

I know you want to. You wouldn't be here otherwise. I have the blueprint. So let's do this.

It's time to take your next step as a fitness professional.

Wait, what was the first step?

You've come to this book to learn about online training. Before you do that, however, we should talk about how you got here. The vast majority of online trainers started out as one-on-one personal trainers who reached a certain point of success but plateaued. Some became gym owners and others decided that wasn't for them. In both situations, they're looking for the next level in their career, to earn more money and freedom while doing what they love.

I hope that's you, because if you haven't spent any time working one-on-one with in-person clients, you're not ready for this book.

I'm a realistic guy and believe it's not just important, but crucial for all trainers to get in-person experience for a minimum of a year before starting online training. You can probably make the business work, but I'd bet you won't do a good enough job with your clients. If you can't deliver results, no amount of marketing will help you.

Training people online demands a much more proactive

approach. It requires you to anticipate the problems a client is likely to have, and do what you can to prevent them. Why? You can't react as well to things that may happen during their training.

Think of it this way: It's like trying your luck on the Olympic diving platform when you've never so much as jumped off the one-meter springboard at your local rec center. Sure, you might figure out a thing or two on the way down, but imagine the pain if you don't. One belly flop from 10 meters will ensure you never try anything that scary again.

Training clients in person is the equivalent of figuring things out on that low board before you take your chances on the platform. Do that for a solid one to three years, and you'll be ready for the next step toward freedom.

What online training *isn't*

You've no doubt seen and heard about all the juicy financial possibilities of online training. One of my goals with the *Wealthy Fit Pro Guides* is to be honest and transparent with you at all times, so you should know up front that I don't view online training as a way to magically make boatloads of cash with very little work.

If only, right?

In the past, people have accused me of turning online training into a commodity, just another offering that has you trading dollars per hour similar to a gym. That's not even close to the truth. I view online training as a way to make life better for *even more* clients, people who might not engage with a professional coach otherwise. For them, it's nothing but positives: more convenient, potentially cheaper, and just as beneficial as in-person. It benefits you, too. I think every fit pro should have an online component. It is a tool to fight back against the (sometimes) abusive fitness industry. Online training can be a fantastic path to whatever you want to do in the industry, and to the kind of life you want outside of it. But, as you'll soon see, it doesn't have to be all you do. It creates space for you to explore multiple options.

Sure, you can scale it to make tons of money. And maybe that will come later. Or maybe you'll write a book. Maybe you'll be happy just making a few thousand more each month because that means you have more time for your spouse/partner/kids/family/ church/golf league. Or maybe you want to start a gym and build up some bottom-line revenue before opening your doors to give your facility a better chance.*

I don't know what freedom means to you, but I do know two things:

---

* *Just like Online Trainer Academy graduate Malcolm Wilson. He wanted to open a gym but had just become a dad and was working 60-hour weeks. He also wanted to be with his family during this magical time. He swapped out long days in the gym for 10 hours a week training in-home and five hours training online. Then, a year later, he founded Level Up Fitness, his gym in Stratford, Connecticut (read Malcolm's story here:* **onlinetrainer.com/malcolm**).

1. "Happy" is a nebulous term that means something different for everybody, and...
2. Making six figures, while it sounds nice, is a vague, meaningless goal that doesn't really contribute to happiness.

Naturally, if you ask people what they want in life, many will say "to get rich!" Most would prefer happiness, however, and the two are not the same. The more researchers study happiness, the less we understand about it. But a few things are pretty certain:

—As long as our basic needs and loved ones are taken care of, money has almost nothing to do with it. In 2010, in the U.S., $75,000 a year was the magic number.* It's probably a bit more now, but even that number is arbitrary because it really depends on where you live. It usually takes less to live comfortably in a small town, for example, and *lots* more if you live in a big city like New York or San Francisco.

—Maintaining a sense of purpose throughout life leads to fulfillment and longevity. In the now-famous studies of Blue Zones, the areas of the world where people live the longest, a sense of purpose is one of the

----

* *The study, performed by Nobel Prize-winning economists at Princeton University, was called "High income improves evaluation of life but not emotional well-being." Since 2010 the results have held up, with one exception. That was a 2017 Harvard study, which found increased levels of emotional well-being in people who have more than $10 million, as long as they earned it (it wasn't inherited, in other words). Interestingly, the one thing these decamillionaires do that makes them happier is give their money away.*

commonalities for folks living past 100.*

—We overestimate both the intensity and duration of a positive emotional response after buying something (a new car, for example). As Catherine Sanderson, a psychology professor at Amherst, explained in a 2017 *Time* magazine article, "We always think if we just had a little bit more money, we'd be happier. But when we get there, we're not." Our enjoyment of new material things lasts about two weeks. After that, the emotional response withers and it just becomes another thing. Researchers refer to this as either "hedonic adaptation" or "impact bias." There are a few ways to maximize the happiness results you get from a dollar spent. For example:

Choose experiences over material goods. Retail therapy makes it too easy to get on the hedonic treadmill. Invest in experiences — and the memories they produce — especially with loved ones.**

Buy many small pleasures. Dollar for dollar, you'll get less satisfaction from one big purchase compared to a series of smaller ones (like multiple nights or weekends away versus a single vacation).

---

* *I've lived in Nosara, Costa Rica, near Playa Pelada and Playa Guiones beaches, right smack in one of those Blue Zones called the Nicoya Peninsula, and I've seen how residents do their thing. Retirement isn't really a concept there. The elderly are revered, and nobody stops moving. The only people vegging out on the beach are the gringos on vacation trying to get away from their lives. Makes a guy think.*

** *Interestingly, even negative experiences lead to higher levels of emotional well-being than material goods because of our fondness for retelling stories about how bad something was.*

Pay now, consume later. Anticipating a future event is often more enjoyable than the event itself. Paying in full up front is better than making small payments.

Surround yourself with community, family, and friends. Daily social contacts are a big predictor of your emotional well-being.

Maximize the things you must do every day. You have to eat and sleep. Make them as pleasurable as you possibly can (an expensive mattress is a great investment).

READ THIS, BE HAPPIER

Learning what leads to happiness is not a requirement for online training, of course, but it's just about the most important thing you could ever know. If you want to do more reading on the subject, Harvard professor Daniel Gilbert has done brilliant research on it. I recommend:

—His book, Stumbling on Happiness.

—A study called "If Money Doesn't Make You Happy Then You Probably Aren't Spending It Right."

—And a 2003 New York Times *piece called "The Futile Pursuit of Happiness," based on his work. This is one of my all-time favorite essays.*

While this is a business development book, I'd be doing you a disservice if I just talked numbers. If you don't know what kind of life you want, you can't begin to build a business plan. How much money you need to make differs between each person and, as you'll soon see, if you want to carve out your own ideal business and life, then it drives your business decisions.

Notice that I called this series the *Wealthy Fit Pro's Guides* and not the *Rich Fit Pro's Guides* or the *Six-Figure Fit Pro Formula.** Making more money isn't the end goal. Money is a tool. Happiness, or better yet, emotional well-being, is the goal, and the amount of money you need to achieve it is different from what I or anybody else needs.

The process starts with taking back control. Online training helps you do that. From there, if you set the right plan with the blueprint I'm laying out here, you'll have the freedom to attain the wealth you need to be happy.

Control -> freedom -> wealth -> happiness

Earlier I mentioned trainers need one to three years' experience coaching people in person before expanding online. That's not some random number I picked out of a towel bin. Yes, it's about getting valuable training

---

* *That's some super-sweet alliteration, though.*

experience, but there's more to it. Consider the following:

Training clients while working for a gym leaves you exhausted. Why? You're not in control. It's a responsive environment where you're at the mercy of everything from the attitudes of the other trainers to the daily mood of the gym owner. And your clients' schedules. And the weather. And traffic. And just about any other outside forces that take swipes at you.

Again: *You're not in control.*

All good trainers reach a point, usually about — ta-da! — one to three years into their careers, where they need to make more money in less time with a better schedule. Around this same time a trainer has worked with enough in-person clients to be reasonably adept at predicting what's going to happen before it happens and how a client will respond to a program. That, and they've built a foundation of clients, case studies, and the beginnings of a reputation.

Becoming a great online trainer requires a different, parallel skillset than working in person. In a gym you can respond and adapt to a client in real time. Online not so much. Doing a good job online requires you to anticipate issues before they arise and navigate around them. We'll cover this in much more detail later in this guide.

So, for all of the above reasons, online training is not the first step. It's the next step — the transition. It bridges the gap by helping you take back control and thrust your career forward.

How do you start?

That's what this book is for. After working with thousands of students in 79 countries (see sidebar) in my Online Trainer Academy (OTA), the world's first certification program for online trainers,* I can claim some expertise. The Wealthy Fit Pro's Guide to Online Training will give you that basic blueprint you need to take your next step.

But let's talk about a few things here before we dive in. It's critical for you to have the right mindset.

I know you'll be fired up to do a hundred things at once to make this new life happen. You'll be nervous. You'll think you know what to do, or what you *want* to do, but you'll be just unsure enough that you don't stick the first few landings. When faced with a (sometimes scary) transition with a host of unknowns like moving to online training, you can do specific things to seize and maintain control of your situation. My advice:

—Start simple, go slow, and build a foundation. The number of clients needed will be different for everybody and pricing is a complicated topic we'll soon

---

* Not only is OTA the first-ever certification for online trainers, it also boasts the seminal textbook on the subject, The Fundamentals of Online Training, and doubles as a business development course with unlimited lifetime mentorship. We also include an ironclad 10-year guarantee. If you're already sold, go to theptdc.com/ota to enroll.

WE'RE EVERYWHERE!

The Online Trainer Academy teaches students from these countries and proves you can live anywhere and run a terrific online training business.

Algeria	France	Norway
Afghanistan	Germany	Pakistan
Australia	Guatemala	Panama
Austria	Haiti	Peru
Bahrain	Hungary	Philippines
Bangladesh	Iceland	Poland
Barbados	India	Portugal
Belgium	Indonesia	Qatar
Belize	Ireland	Romania
Bermuda	Israel	Russia
Bolivia	Italy	South Africa
Brazil	Jamaica	Scotland
Brunei	Japan	Serbia
Bulgaria	Kenya	Singapore
Burma	Korea	Slovakia
Canada	Kuwait	Slovenia
Chile	Latvia	Spain
China	Lithuania	Sweden
Costa Rica	Luxembourg	Switzerland
Croatia	Macedonia	Taiwan
Cyprus	Malaysia	Thailand
Czech Republic	Mauritius	Turkey
Denmark	Mexico	U.A.E.
Egpyt	Netherlands	Wales
England	New Zealand	Zimbabwe
Estonia	Nicaragua	
Finland	Northern Ireland	

cover. Starting out, five to 10 clients is usually enough. This lets you wade into the pool without getting in over your head (full submersion comes later).

And look how well it can work: 10 clients at $200 a month is an extra $2,000 per month or $24,000 per year, more than enough to allow you to cut loose in-person clients you don't jell with or who don't fit into a tight schedule.

Time, aside from money, is the first serious benefit of online training. The total number of hours you put in might not change much. (Usually it's less depending on how you structure things. We'll talk about support systems in a bit). The difference is you're now in control of your schedule. You decide when you work.

—Next thing: Did I mention start simple, go slow? Blocking off your schedule better will open up more time to develop all the other things that could make you money and raise your professional profile. Better marketing opportunities. Creating new products. Firing on that book you've always dreamed of writing.

You'll be tempted to take on *everything*. Respect the power of high-yield activities within your new schedule, but also respect how much you'll be able to accomplish and still serve your clients well (we guide our OTA students with two principles. The second is to always ask yourself, "What would this look like if it were easy?").

It sounds nice to write an ebook and sell thousands of

copies passively. In theory, developing a membership program where you take on 50, 100, or hundreds of clients with variations of templates and online group support sounds great. All of these things are very real possibilities, but none of them comes first.

What comes first?

Decide what you really, truly want from this career progression. As your newfound scheduling freedom becomes real, you now have room to think, breathe, and work. And that, my friend, is where the magic happens. It allows you to be methodical. Don't start an avalanche of projects you can't manage and will end up rushing through just to say you got them done.

I'm all about simplification and focus. Building an online fitness business, just like building a body, is a process. You wouldn't do a pistol squat with a k-bell before learning how to sit on a chair, would you? Unfortunately, many fail because they disrespect the process.

This book will walk you through that process. As you learn more, decide whether you want to take on more online clients, write a book, or use the extra time that's resulted in a more structured schedule to volunteer, travel, spend more time with your family, or develop the in-depth marketing funnels required to make significant money selling your wares.

Decide.

My definition of wealth is synonymous with freedom. Freedom lets me dictate my own life. It lets me spend mornings and lunch chasing my toddler son.* It lets me travel the world for months at a stretch and live as a native in amazing places. Costa Rica, Hawaii, Thailand, Mexico, Montenegro, Greece. I live the life I want.

But don't take it from me. So many graduates of my Online Trainer Academy are living their dreams.

Daniel Lopez wanted to sing opera. Making a living is difficult as a performer, so he became a trainer and put his opera career on hold. Online training has allowed him to quit his in-person training and return to his true love. He performs around the world and has even landed movie roles (read his story here: **onlinetrainer. com/daniel**).

Keep reading. You'll hear even more stories and crucial business advice from OTA grads throughout the book. They inspire me every day, so let them inspire you, too.

Your definition of wealth is probably different from mine or Daniel's but one thing I do know: When you really think about, it has nothing to do with becoming a "six-figure trainer."

Whatever your definition is, it comes to life here. It's your turn to challenge the norms. The next step is online training, so let's take it together.

—Coach Jon

---

* Speaking of which, why did nobody tell me that friggin' two-year-olds were so fast? I feel like I'm running wind sprints multiple times a day wondering where the heck this kid gets his energy.

CHAPTER 1

The Foundation of a Successful Online Trainer

By Alex Cartmill

"While there's money to be made in this industry, if you're in it for the money, the work and road ahead will seem grueling. If you're here because you love what you do, the money will find you."

—Tim Henriques

We want online training to be the best possible fit for you. That's why you need to know something up front: Online training isn't magic.

It's full of possibilities. It can change your life. But you can't wave a wand, call yourself an online trainer, and solve all your problems. Here, at the beginning, it's critical for you to understand how online training does, or doesn't, align with your goals and personality. Only then can you decide if it makes sense for you.

I manage a team of Online Trainer Academy coaches and mentors who interact daily with our thousands of students. Over the course of a given day we'll have a dozen live chats, 10 phone calls, and 30-plus emails. That's a massive amount of interaction with online trainers hustling in every conceivable pocket of the industry. As a result, over time, we've been able to track who succeeds and who fails, what works and what doesn't.

In this chapter, I'll highlight a typical (successful!) trainer's traits and what clients thrive in this environment. We'll discuss your experience, motivation, what kind of clients you prefer, how well they might do with a remote coach, and your definition of freedom. Or, better said, how you envision living your perfect day.*

Don't worry. Even if you read a few things in here that make you think, *Oh crap, that really isn't me*, or *I don't have the experience*, or *Maybe I'm wasting my time*, please keep reading. People grow into roles and blossom. Just because your background may not scream "online training is my destiny!" today doesn't mean you can't

---

* *On my perfect day I get to take my dog, Charlie, out for lots of walks. He's getting bigger though. So he kind of walks me these days.*

learn what you need to become a great digital coach.

And that, friends, is why we say online training isn't magic. It's work, but worth the effort.

Let's talk about the foundation of a successful online trainer.

Experience

In the intro, Coach Jon mentioned you need one to three years' experience before trying online training. Let's dig deeper into that so you have a full understanding why.

The main difference between training someone in person and online is immediacy. In person, you watch them train, coach them as they go, and offer advice or answer questions in real time. When you say, "I'm here for you," you literally are.

Online? Not so much. Yes, you interact, but you're remote. That's why training people online requires a deeper understanding of the entire process. You'll give a client your program, but you won't be there to answer a question while she does it. You have to have the know-how to proactively anticipate what *may* happen and side-step problems before they occur.

Example: Let's say you work with a client in person who sits at a desk all day. During an upper-body pressing movement, she says, "I feel this pinching in my shoulder." Because you're right there, you can stop the movement, talk to her about what it feels like, and adjust as needed.

Now take this interaction online. She may feel the pinching during her workout, but she won't bring it up until afterward. Meanwhile, she may have injured herself because she wanted to power through the pain and finish her reps. *That should never happen.* If you're working with that deskbound client online, you should already know to avoid programming pronated upper-body pressing movements because they might cause discomfort.

You and I both know, as professionals, that every body is different. I think we'd also agree there are some commonalities among demographics. Does every desk jockey have to avoid pronated pressing? Absolutely not. Some might be blessed with more space in their glenohumeral joint. But this is where online differs from in-person. You have to categorize people based on experience and best guesses, and program around it.

Always ask yourself: Is there a potentially safer alternative that still achieves the same training goal? If so, plug it in proactively. That's what makes a great online coach.

If you've trained this type of clientele before, you're probably nodding your head, thinking what I just said was obvious. If you've never trained this clientele, however, you might be wondering what I'm talking about. And that's my entire point.

Effective online trainers only take on clients in situations they're familiar with. This is why in-person experience is necessary to do a good job online. There are way too many coaching nuances you can only learn in person.

There's more. Good experience isn't just about programming. A bunch of other important aspects of the job are amplified in a remote environment: Customer support, client accountability, operating systems, outsourcing work, and more.*

Think of your approach to online training like the tagline from those Farmer's Insurance commercials: "We know a thing or two because we've seen a thing or two." You need that experience to keep online clients happy, safe, and thriving.

Motives

I know all about the "allure" of online training. Come on, you know what I'm talking about. The joys of coaching clients from your laptop while lounging on the beach sipping a mai tai. The beach and type of drink may change from coach to coach, but the daydream is the same.

Let's be frank: If working fewer hours and posting pictures of your sandy toes are your driving forces for

---

* A smile does wonders in person. An emoji smile doesn't quite have the same effect. Text messages and emails can easily be taken the wrong way if they aren't written carefully and, without the benefit of a smile, could get you in trouble.

working online, you'll hop off this train as soon as the going gets tough. And it will get tough. Will you get going?

Before you take your game online, consider your motives.

The most successful online trainers are driven by one, or both, of the following:

1. A need to serve

Successful online trainers put their clients first. They don't do it out of a sense of duty. They feel genuine joy helping others. It's part of their DNA and why they got into personal training in the first place. Becoming an online trainer because you think it will be easier and more lucrative will lead you down a long, frustrating path.

Yes, online training will allow you the freedom to work on your own schedule, and there's a good chance to boost your income. But if money is the only thing pushing you forward, you'll come up short with your clients. You'll cut corners. You'll get a lousy reputation. And even if you make the money you want, you'll eventually give up because the purpose and fulfillment that we all crave isn't there.

The truth is counterintuitive, but it's true all the same: The trainers driven by love and appreciation for the work and a passion for helping others (and who have a baseline understanding of business development and marketing) end up with the most money. Why? Clients will always hire them, and fellow fit pros will always support them.

2. A desire for a more balanced and fulfilling life

Budding trainers are told they can't make a living in this industry without working 12-hour days and to accept that norm without challenging it. Those trainers burn out because they're doomed for mediocrity off the bat. It takes guts to challenge this norm, but it's the only way upward.

Consider Francis McCabe, an Online Trainer Academy graduate from Belfast, Ireland and owner of Precision Online Coaching: Between his full-time job at the fire department and part-time gig as a personal trainer, Francis started his days at 6 a.m. and staggered home at 9:30 p.m., only to go to bed to do it all again the next day. He tolerated this schedule for a while, but once Francis became a dad he vowed to spend more time with his family.

Now a typical day looks very different for Francis. He works his online business for several hours in the morning, enjoys a home workout, takes a walk with his daughter and their dogs, has lunch with his daughter, and spends some time reading on personal development in the afternoon (read Francis' full story here: **onlinetrainer.com/francis**).

And no, Francis isn't making millions. He's making what he needs to sustain his ideal lifestyle and spend ample time with his family. That's what matters.

The right niche

Oh, trainers do love their niches. Not familiar with the term? A niche is a specialized area of expertise a trainer (a) loves working in, (b) gets really good at, and (c) eventually becomes a known authority and in-demand talent.

OTA students have had success in a plethora of niches: older clients, kids, recreational athletes, various interest groups, different professions, you name it. There are a lot of options, and no inherently best one.

Most niche clients will succeed online, but not all. Let's talk about that here.

The following three populations probably *shouldn't* be trained online. If you enjoy training in one of these niches and aspire to take your business online, be careful. As with anything, there are exceptions to these rules and ultimately you'll have to be the judge. If you feel like you can get the results that a client deserves, then take him on. But understand that OTA students have consistently experienced difficulties working within these niches:

- *Clients in any kind of rehabilitative environment.* When continual testing and fine-tuning is required, there really is no substitute for in-person.

- *High-performance athletes.* When the difference

between winning and losing is a fraction of a second, every rep matters. It's brutal trying to coach from a distance at that level.

- *Clients who have never exercised before.* A new client doesn't just need to be taught proper form. He or she needs to be taught how to "feel" movement. Additionally, even a motivated client may still have reservations based on fear, uncertainty, and a general hesitation to start something new. In-person is the best option here.

Enjoyment

Online training isn't right for every client and it's certainly not right for every trainer. Even though it's appealing on paper, the day-to-day realities of the job might become too much if you're the wrong personality for it. Don't let the promise of more freedom and more money blind you.

John Berardi, founder of Precision Nutrition, offered a good litmus test to our OTA students a few years back. Ask yourself a simple question: "Where do I want my butt to be throughout the day?"

Extroverted people may want to reconsider full-time online training. If you're energized in the gym and feel downtrodden the second you have to turn on your computer, well, you might not be online trainer material.

A viable compromise: Go hybrid. A lot of folks work

well with a mix of online and in-person (most of our OTA students maintain a gym-based client list, and we'll talk in more detail about this later).

While our refund rate is low in the Academy (about two percent), half of those former students simply realized online training wasn't for them. They tried it, got their first few clients, and decided they wanted to be around people all the time. That's cool. We happily refunded their tuition. Successful, fulfilled students are our goal.

Make sure fulfillment is *your* priority as you make your way through this book and discover what online training can deliver.

THE TAKEAWAY

Transitioning to online training isn't automatic. It has to align with your goals and personality. Make sure you have the proper foundational experience and genuine motivation, and understand what kind of clients have the best success training with a remote coach. It's okay if you realize that online training isn't a good fit.

Bonus: Get Your Take Action Checklist Now

We're about to get into all of the bits and pieces that make up a stellar online training business. To help keep you organized, we've put together a handy checklist with pages in this book for reference.

Go to **www.theptdc.com/checklist** to get yours now so you can fill it in as you go.

CHAPTER 2

Choose Your Online Business Model

> *"People are always looking for the single magic bullet that will totally change everything. There is no single magic bullet."*
>
> —Temple Grandin

If life were one size fits all, it would be so much easier. And so boring.

Online training is the same way. You can go in any number of directions. Several business models exist, and the right model in the right person's wheelhouse can be gold. And you can probably guess what the wrong model for the wrong person produces. So let's jump right in: *What kind of online training business model do you want?*

Don't worry, we'll give you the rundown, the pros

and cons, and the pitfalls, and describe what kind of personalities tend to thrive in each. But even with all that, you're the one best judge of what may or may not work for you. And guess what? Here's a little-known secret: You can change your mind. You can pivot. You can adapt. You can, dare we say it, *have fun* with the process of discovery. Too many people forget that part.

Let's do this.

The three online training business models

The first thing you need to know: None of these models are inherently right or wrong. None of them are created equal, either, and each will result in a different business structure. You may already have an idea of what kind of business you want to build based on things you've read or other operations you've seen (successful trainers are highly visible folks, after all). For now, put aside what you think you know. You need to understand how each model works before you decide.

The three models are:

1. **One to Many.** One trainer works simultaneously with 50-plus clients who pay lower fees, usually through a membership platform.
2. **High-Ticket Coaching.** One trainer works with a very small group of clients who pay big fees.
3. **One to a Few.** One trainer works with five to 30 clients and charges anywhere from $100 to $500 per month.

Those first two models sound appealing. One lets you scale up, the other delivers high margins. Before you jump in, however, a myriad of problems hide in the shadows of both.

One too many problems

The first model forces you to...

Compete on price. You'll cater to consumers looking for the cheapest product, which means they may not be the most dedicated clients. And because your goal is to get as many clients through the door as possible, you'll unintentionally devalue some important things: It'll be far more challenging to differentiate yourself through your services, or take the time to build a network of genuine relationships with people who will pay a higher fee because they know, like, and trust you.

Manage a lot of customers. That means a larger administrative burden. Sterling customer service is *crucial* in our industry, and it's mutually exclusive from your client total. Why? Whether you have five or 500, poor customer service will crush your reputation and hamper growth. Now imagine the challenge of managing 500 clients versus five. Big numbers require that much more time, energy, and people.

De-emphasize the personal touch. Have you heard the phrase, "People buy trainers, not training?" I bet you have, and it's too important to ignore. You see, your best clients, the ones who will fuel your business for years to come through repeat business and word of mouth, buy into You the Human as well as You the Expert. Here you're spreading yourself too thin to provide that personal touch.

This model can work for someone who really knows how to market and manage a big operation. Of course, that requires a team of full-time marketers and a high ad budget to make it flourish. If that's you, fine, but understand you'll be a marketer, not a trainer. That's why it's not for us, and we don't teach it at the Online Trainer Academy.

High ticket = high risk

I get the appeal of working with affluent clients who pay country club prices for your services. But you gotta know: Big price tags mean big expectations. Are you up for that?

Here's what I mean: It's your job to make an affluent client's health and fitness as seamless and easy for them as possible. An "exclusive" feel is part of the package. That means catering to their schedule, location, and demands. You have to be there for them. Not only can this cost a chunk of *your* money and time to accommodate, the grind can be unrealistic for a trainer with a family or other obligations.

Oh, and let's talk about the risk. This model is fragile. Like, butterfly-wing fragile. If you have five clients and one bails, you've just lost 20 percent of your revenue overnight.

That gives each client an incredible amount of power over you and your business. Plus, recruiting new clients requires a strong connection and pre-established trust, so replacing that lost client can be a long process.

Some people make this model work and enjoy it. But it breaks too easily, and as a result, it's not for us and we don't teach it at OTA.

Introducing: the incredible, gloriously unsexy, stable, and very realistic One to a Few model

We teach this model at the OTA and a lot of grads have made it the foundation of their businesses. It's a realistic and stable path built on core truths, not surface-level techniques, for those fed up with sensationalistic promises. It doesn't require advanced marketing, tech savvy, paid advertising, costly software, or even a website to get started.

What it's not? Fast. If you're less patient, this model probably isn't for you. But what it lacks in speed it makes up for in reliability. Simply put, this model is accessible to every trainer — no matter your background, marketing acumen, technical know-how, or anything else.

And yes, it's difficult to make millions with it, but you will make more than you make now, and do it on your own schedule. From there, you decide what comes next. Some fit pros decide to invest in additional marketing and scale their revenue significantly, while others decide they're content. That's called freedom.

You don't see this model publicized often because it's not sexy to sell, and requires you to play the long game. You'll likely notice, on the flip side, a plethora of coaches and mentors selling the high-ticket approach to dramatically and quickly increase your income, and making it look easy. But if it were that easy to charge thousands per month per client and make hundreds of thousands of dollars with very little effort... don't you think everybody would be doing it?

None of these approaches are inherently right or wrong, but they make you spend your time and money in different places and have different levels of risk. It's important to understand that.

The great snowball fight

To help illustrate the fundamental differences in One to a Few compared to, say, High Ticket, imagine a snowball fight.

Our method is akin to a patient warrior taking her time, creating a big pyramid of snowballs before even thinking of firing a shot. A High Ticket approach would have you make one big honking snowball and launch it immediately.

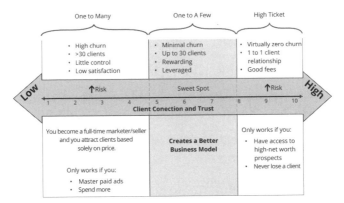

This graph illustrates the various risks between the three online business models. The One to Many model is risky on the low end of the "Connection and Trust" scale because of high churn and a need for endless marketing. The High Ticket model is risky on the high side of the scale because your business can be disrupted by just one "personal connection" client leaving. The One to a Few model is the least risky because you land right in the sweet spot: a healthy number of clients, the ability to deliver a personal touch to every service you offer, and a better work-life balance (and income!).

The big snowball will usually miss. But if it hits, hey, it's high-impact. BOOM.

If you only consider the first half of the fight, you might think the person making lots of snowballs will lose. But stick around for the second half and she's sitting there with a pile of snowballs ready for anything while the High Ticket snowballer has to start over from scratch after each throw.

You get the idea. Yes, each plan can work if you bring the right resources, but it's easier to think of One to a Few as the smart middle ground between all possibilities. Not too many clients, each paying a slight premium compared to the discount model. And you remove most of the downside risks of the other two models. For example:

- Losing a client won't cripple your business.
- You'll always have a manageable number of clients, which makes good customer service simpler.
- You can concentrate on client results and building a great reputation.
- You can charge what you're worth.
- You can do it on your own schedule.

The One to a Few approach is our chosen method because it's virtually guaranteed (and if you decide to enroll in the Online Trainer Academy at some point, then it's 100 percent guaranteed because we'll happily give you your money back if it doesn't work; but we know it will).

A great engineer takes pride in building a machine that will run for a long time without needing constant tweaks. If you want to build a fitness business that works for years to come, build it on a solid foundation.

Check out some other options

Now let's talk about models that exist within those big three models. This section cuts right to the style of training you prefer, as each of the following options can be applied to any primary model.

Hybrid Training

Hybrid training combines face-to-face and online training. You now charge two fees:

- Regular in-person session fee.

- A monthly "performance plan" fee for managing your online clients' programming.

While you're online, think of yourself not as a trainer who counts sets and reps, but as a concierge service in charge of your clients' preventive health.

Benefits:

- You create a reliable secondary income stream while still working at a gym.

- It's an easy way to transition from in-person to online training, without the pressure of needing the new business to provide all your income.

- It gives clients a more flexible and cost-effective option besides training face-to-face.

- You can offer a client what they need, when they need it.*

Drawbacks:

---

* When a client begins training with you, they'll likely need more in-person time. As their training progresses, odds are they'll need to see you less. Meanwhile, clients may want increased in-person service in preparation for an upcoming event like a wedding or vacation. The hybrid training model we developed back in 2013 has become our most popular because it removes all business constraints from training, allowing a client's fitness goals to dictate how the business operates. That's a big win on all sides.

- You'll be limited by location, as you'll still meet with clients on a semi-regular basis.

- Requires explanation, and varying from "the norms" can be a hard(er) sell to a client. — Even if you don't remove the in-person element completely, you're still prisoner to whatever existing perceptions your clients have about what they should and shouldn't pay for.

This may be right for you if:

- You want to transition online but not abandon in-person completely.

- You want to expand your income streams.

- You have clients who don't need you there 100 percent of the time, but still need some hands-on work.

With the Online Trainer Academy's lessons, strategies, and scripts, Daniel Lona was able to add Lean and Confident, his online nutrition coaching program, to his existing business in Chicago to create a secondary stream of income and give himself more flexibility with his schedule. He also does private one-on-one training (kettlebells are his specialty).

"Since last year, I've been making online nutrition coaching a major part of my business," he says, "and this helps me be a far better coach to my clients by offering them a higher standard of service. (Creating an awesome experience in the form of an online business ain't exactly intuitive, ya know!)" Read his story here: **onlinetrainer.com/daniel-lona.**

Individualized Online Coaching

Here you take the one-on-one care you provide your in-person clients and transfer it online.

Of course, the structure of coaching will vary, but this type of foundation generally includes two to three different packages that vary in length and level of support. You'll provide a customized program specific to a client's goals, have regular check-ins, email support, and accountability boosters, and provide the same quality and care you would in person.

Benefits:

- Location is no longer a factor. You can work with clients anywhere in the world.
- It's usually more cost-effective for the client than in-person training.
- You have the ability to help more clients than in-person training allows.
- You work your own schedule.

Drawbacks:

- You won't be able to take on as many clients as you would with full-on group training.
- You have to be comfortable sitting at a computer for long stretches.

This may be right for you if:

- You're transitioning out of training in-person at the gym.
- You plan to work with a similar clientele, or even transition some of your in-person clients, online.

Michael Bieter, an OTA grad and founder of Pillar Coaching Services in Des Moines, Iowa, is a great example of how to build a one-on-one coaching business online.

Mike knew early on that the fitness industry was his calling. By 12th grade, Mike was working in the high school gym and got his fitness certification at just 18 years old. He wasted no time putting it to use and got a job in a gym where he expanded on his fitness knowledge and learned about nutrition. Soon he was managing large, highly profitable facilities.

Unfortunately, at a certain point, the rose-colored glasses had to come off. Mike explains, "I disagreed with the management a lot. We had different values. The approach seemed to be 'turn 'em and burn 'em.' Get their money and move on. I didn't agree with the way they were dieting the clients either. It wasn't right to me."

Mike enrolled in the Online Trainer Academy, implemented the material immediately, and soon after signed 18 new clients. He now works with 80 to 100 clients himself and has hired another coach who works with 30 to 40 at a time. Now Mike manages his day in a way that works for him, allowing him to serve his clients well. He has his freedom back and, most important for him, a new chance to live his values. Read his story here: **onlinetrainer.com/michael.**

Online Group Training

Forming a group allows you to offer a more cost-effective program while individualizing your templates for each client. The major difference between group training and one-on-one is that you scale your support systems to offer less individual attention while still "being there" for each person as needed.

Benefits:

- You can take on more clients than with one-on-one coaching.

- It's more cost-effective for you and your clients.

Drawbacks:

- It's not as involved as one-on-one coaching or individual transformations.

- You'll need to manage and offer customer service to a higher number of clients.

- Client turnover is generally higher.

- Ongoing marketing is required to make up for lost clients and fuel growth.

This may be right for you if:

- You want to offer a more cost-effective structure and serve a large audience.

- You have the ability to generate ample leads.

- You're good at building systems to help you juggle a lot of moving parts.

OTA graduate Terrell Baldock from Ontario, Canada, uses group coaching in her business, Mom's Fitness Boutique, aimed at new moms.

Terrell became a personal trainer by fairly traditional means: She got her certification and started at a big box gym. The longer she worked there, however, the less happy she became. "I was told it was a good thing to make prospective clients cry during a consultation," she says, "because they'd be more likely to buy."

That values mismatch widened as Terrell got pregnant and had her first child. She realized the gym's expectations and rigid schedules didn't allow for the flexibility a new mom requires — especially one struggling with severe postpartum depression, as was the case for Terrell.

"I wouldn't sleep for two or three days, I was suffering from adrenal fatigue," she recalls. "It was bad. But I couldn't get anyone to cover my shift."

At the same time, Terrell noticed a huge gap in service: Prenatal and postpartum needs were not being met in a traditional training environment. She decided to use her first-hand experience to bridge that gap. Terrell went from two clients to almost 30 in just five months. And the clients keep coming. In fact, she's looking to hire a new trainer to help her keep up with demand. Read her story here: **onlinetrainer.com/terrell.**

Group Transformation Programs

A transformation program is not all that different from a regular online training package, but it typically promotes a specific goal with a specific timeline. Think, "lose eight pounds in 30 days." You'll need a curriculum and a program template for the specified time of your challenge. The key to success with this method is marketing your transformation program to one specific population, with one specific goal ("Slim down for wedding season," for example).

Benefits:

- A lot of clients come through your online "door" at once.

- It's more cost effective for you and your clients.

- Once you get this system running, you can turn it off and on whenever you like.

- With the right systems, many of the online processes can be automated and scaled.

- You sell the benefit of the transformation, making marketing easier.

Drawbacks:

- Programming isn't as individualized as one-on-one coaching.

- With a larger number of clients, it's easy to skimp on the care and attention each client deserves. Good customer service systems are a must.

- Programming is short-term, potentially leading to higher client turnover. You'll have to fill vacant slots each session, which can be challenging.

- You need to choose clients carefully. A group is only as strong as its weakest link, and a destructive member can bring everyone down.

This may be right for you if:

- You have the ability to generate ample leads.

- You're good at building systems to help you juggle a lot of moving parts at once.

OTA grad Gil Mesina from Toronto, Ontario, utilizes group transformation programs in his business, Mighty Transformation.

Gil's setup has three different levels, each building off the last. For instance, clients have to complete his first-tier Genesis program before they can enroll in his second-tier Elevation program. While Gil will allow someone to join a higher-tier group through an application process if they're a good fit, this structure has helped him build ongoing accountability and rapport with every client. It's also helped him ensure the service he's providing, although on a group level, is well-suited for each individual.

Gil opens up his group transformation programs to new clients every 12 weeks, after the previous group finishes up, and repeats the process every three months. Read Gil's story here: **onlinetrainer.com/gil.**

Live Stream Workouts

This is a total tech takeover: You watch your client's workout live via video. This can be an effective route for clients who prefer, or would benefit from, their coach's immediate presence (even if the coach is halfway around the world). This can work well for individuals and group environments, and for any activity — you can be there to offer corrections and support for yoga, a HIIT workout, or anything in between. Some coaches perform the workout right along with their clients.

Additionally, live stream workouts don't have to comprise 100 percent of your client's workouts. They can be used intermittently to check in on your client's movement patterns or even for the occasional group workout with all of your clients to have a little fun and strengthen relationships.

Benefits:

- You're able to "be" with your clients while they work out. Great for analyzing technique and answering questions on the spot.

- Increases accountability and adherence, as it's less likely a client will skip a workout.

Drawbacks:

- Time commitment is greater for each client.

- You have less control over your schedule. Both coach and client must find a time to "meet."

- You're limited in the number of clients you can take on at one time.

- If your clients go to a gym, you may run into problems with them filming inside. A conversation with gym management may be required.

This may be right for you if:

- You want to work with clientele who need a more "hands-on" environment where technique can be corrected instantly.

- You want to help online clientele struggling with adherence and consistency.

- Your online clients still want their coach to be with them during workouts.

Online Trainer Academy grad Arpita Boyd utilizes live stream coaching in her online coaching business, Mind and Body PT. She's originally from India but now travels the world with her family. Arpita has live-streamed client workouts while on a train in India, a mountain in Switzerland, and an island near Croatia.

It's mutually beneficial: Her clients get the structure and presence they need to succeed, and Arpita lives the life she wants. As she says: "Yes, it *is* possible to be on the other side of the world and also nail your technique via online personal training." Read her story here: **onlinetrainer.com/arpita.**

How to choose?

Okay. Based on everything you just read, you have some big decisions to make. As you flip through the options in your head, here's an idea: Move on to the next chapter. Bet it'll be a big help.

THE TAKEAWAY

Which online business model is right for you? It's a big choice — just remember to be honest about what kind of trainer you want to be and what clients will inspire you. No business model is inherently wrong, but certain models will be wrong for you. What feels right?

CHAPTER 3

Build an Unbeatable Business Mindset

"At the end of the day, you are solely responsible for your success and your failure. And the sooner you realize that, you accept that, and integrate that into your work ethic, you will start being successful. As long as you blame others for the reason you aren't where you want to be, you will always be a failure."

— Erin Cummings

Beginners complicate. Experts simplify.

Remember that. Read it, learn it, live it. It's a simple truth that veteran trainers see over and over.

This chapter is all about your mind. You see, your mind messes with you. Maybe you know that already. But if you can improve your business mindset, learn stronger ways to make decisions, you'll improve your chances at success. A big deal, to be sure. And that's why I lead with that statement.

Obviously, you want to execute like an expert, but unfortunately a lot of newer trainers fall back on human instinct, which in this instance shows up as fear, hesitation, and overanalyzing. You might think you're being cautious and intuitive. In reality, you're worrying about the wrong things.

So let's talk about mindset and how to make confident decisions.

What's *really* holding you back?

Don't come down with analysis paralysis. That's a beginner trait. The fact is, most of the decisions you'll have to make are pretty simple. By agonizing over every insignificant dissimilarity of each business component along the way, you put yourself in quicksand that will pull you down every single day, keeping you from moving forward.

So what's going on? And why does this happen to so many trainers? Let's simplify it...

- They don't know what their clients truly need.
- They fear the unknown.

That's pretty much it. Think it through:

What do your clients truly need? Don't mix this up with what *you* think your clients need. Many trainers simply don't understand what stepping stones will lead them to their ultimate goal. As a result, every decision becomes world-hanging-in-the-balance critical in their mind. Every decision seems to require time, and thought, when in reality you should make some decisions quickly and never think about them again. Why? They probably aren't as crucial as you think.

Take one of the most pondered and discussed topics of online training: software.

Every single day we hear, "What online training software is best?" Or, "What's the difference between Software X and Software Y?" when both provide the same essential services. We've seen trainers take months testing out different software, dwelling on every minor discrepancy between them.

Experts simplify, so try this: I.D. three things you need software to do, pick a software that does those things, and never think about it again. Done.

... but wait that's too fast it might not work what if it's the wrong choice what will happen this is crazy you're moving too fast...

Stop. It's just not that big a deal. Will you discover things about the software you chose that bug you? Probably. Will they ruin your business and keep your clients from coming back? Probably not. Again, take the time to understand what you and your clients actually need, and filter all of your decisions through that.*

And if you're already using a software program? Stick with it. Don't even look at other options. What you have is surely good enough, I promise. You've got more important things to focus on.

What are you afraid of? Fear is an irrational response to the unknown, and oftentimes it's that fear of the unknown, of the next step, that forces us into unnecessary analysis. In that regard, fear is very much a choice. Why give it so much power over you?

To drive away fear, define the unknown. In this example, pick the software that has the major qualities you need, and move on. The unknown is now known, and you didn't lose valuable time wandering in the forest, fearful of what will happen next, hoping for an answer, when you have the power to leave anytime you want.

Hey, let's talk money!

Another big issue that affects every decision: The great unknown abyss called income. Yeah, maybe you can outsweat anybody in the gym, but the spectre of money can turn that sweat dead cold. Money's scary stuff.

If you're starting an online training business, how much do you need to make it work? Remember, we're not just talking about subsisting or "muddling through." You're

---

** To make this even easier, we maintain an up-to-date comparison chart of all the major online training software here: **theptdc.com/software.***

going online to make more money than you are right now, and make even more in the future.

That's why, starting out, you have to identify your "freedom number," the monthly income you need to pull in for a sustainable and satisfying life. This number puts your path to success in perspective and shines a light on the unknown. It helps define what's really holding you back, so you can move forward.

Online Trainer Academy graduate Patrick Murphy from Jacksonville, Florida, discovered how realistic his goals were with his business MurphyFit.com after calculating his freedom number:

"When you sit down and honestly, truthfully figure out your freedom number, you realize why it's called that, because it's not as much as you think it is."

With a freedom number of $2,250 per month, Patrick's irrational business fears were put in perspective. Patrick was able to meet his freedom number from online coaching, while also serving as the strength and conditioning coach of the minor league Jacksonville Icemen hockey team.[*]

Calculate your freedom number

The math is wonderfully simple. Start by tallying up the amount of money per month, after taxes, that you require to fulfill your basic needs: rent, food, funds to

---

* As a Canadian, I find it hilarious that they have ice hockey in Florida.

care for dependents (if applicable), and a small amount for extravagance. Figure out what *your* number is. Don't worry about anybody else's.

Now work up what's known as your "continued funds," which is money you make either passively (from investments or maybe book sales) or by doing what you love to do. For the latter, that's money made through other work that you never plan to stop. Example: You still want to train 10 in-person clients along with your new online clientele. Calculate how much you make from those 10 clients each month and there you have your "continued funds."

Now use this formula:

Your freedom number = essentials - continued funds

Your freedom number is crucial because it gives you an earnings target each month. Once you figure out this number, you'll use online training to fill the gap. Hit or surpass the number each month and you're safe and free to pursue riskier or more ambitious strategies that require a lot of development time.

If your freedom number happens to be negative, that's fantastic. You're able to fulfill your basic needs doing the work you love. In turn, you're able to take risks and really build out your online business your way, and not have to rely on it for income. I bet you didn't know this before you did the calculation though, did you?

THREE WHO ARE "FREE"

To show you how vastly different freedom numbers can be for different coaches, three Online Trainer Academy graduates share theirs, along with the reasons why it works for them.

Jameson Skillings

Maine, United States
Freedom number: $1,575
Business name: Skillings Fitness

"My personal training schedule was maxed out. I had already transitioned one-on-one clients to semiprivate and larger strength training groups. I was away from home and working 50 to 70 hours a week. With a toddler at home, I was missing milestones and not spending enough time with my family. It was breaking my heart. I have met or exceeded my freedom goal every month since I graduated from the program and increased my sales by 357 percent in 2018." Read Jameson's story here:
onlinetrainer.com/jameson.

Jason Leenaarts

Ohio, United States
Revolution Fitness and Therapy
Freedom number: $10,000

"My freedom number is an overlap from what it

takes to keep my brick-and-mortar business open, pay my employees, and cover my bills. Anything made above and beyond that number was gravy."

Using OTA principles, Jason was able to meet his freedom number and, as Jason puts it, "take some of the pressure off of me to make sure that everything is perfect." Read Jason's story here: **onlinetrainer.com/jason.**

Shiggi Pakter

London, United Kingdom
Superbodied Performance
Freedom Number: £2,100 (about $2,700)

Shiggi prefers to make her own rules as a part-time online trainer. Her number covers expenses but also includes "£1k extra" a month, which makes room for her multiple interests, most notably her budding DJ career using the moniker NeoPink. "My goal is to only work with clients online. If they want to see me in person, it comes at a premium because otherwise I'm in studios or flying around Europe." Read Shiggi's story here: **onlinetrainer.com/shiggi.**

More tools for an unbeatable mindset

When Thomas Edison worked on some shiny new thing, he'd alert the press before the invention was finished to create a deadline for himself. This put Edison in a position to either take action and justify the excitement he created, or tarnish his trust and reputation. The choice was easy.

That's one way to push yourself to perform, to get your mind out of the way so you can get the job done. We've got a bunch of effective strategies for this, as you'll see in a second, but this is a good one to kick off the section.

Motivate yourself with accountability.
Accountability moves you forward. And who better to hold you accountable than the people you're selling to? Simply announce your new program to your audience X number of weeks before it's done, and start signing people up. This removes your safety net and gives you two options: Take action and deliver, or don't.

It's easy to wait until things are perfect before taking action. The problem is things will never be perfect. This mindset will keep you revising and rethinking and retooling your business to oblivion.

Learn empathy. Empathy keeps your focus where it needs to be: on your clients. Imagine what they're going through, how they feel, what's motivating them. Even the most logical, rational human beings are driven by emotion. Clients will respond to you based on what they feel, not what they (or you) know. Connect on that level and you'll gain their trust. Once you have that, most of the little stuff stops mattering. And speaking of the little stuff...

Never let the micro drive the macro. The vast majority of beginning trainers I communicate with daily are fumbling through and fretting over decisions that are significant to them, but insignificant to their clients.

These are micro decisions that require minimal thought, time, and energy (see software example from earlier). Micro decisions take your focus away from the big picture, from what truly matters.

Macro decisions, on the other hand, serve as the foundation of your business. These are the overarching, fundamental characteristics of your services that will keep clients coming back for years. Macro requires you to step back and view your dilemma through a wider lens. Macro issues truly do matter to your clients, and that's where you need to allocate resources.

What's the difference between a micro and macro problem? Some examples:

Micro	Macro
Business name	Client goals
Color scheme of your website	Client trust
Promoting your certs	Clients receiving value for price
Pushing hot new exercises	Your reputation

See the macro behind all the micro. What if you feel like you have a handle on the macro, but are overwhelmed by wave after wave of micro? Can that even be a thing? Theoretically, yes, but in practice, almost never.

At the Online Trainer Academy, our coaches are trained to see past the superficial and look for the deeper question a student is asking. Defining a root problem almost always provides better results. A lot of the trainers who come to us are stuck, feel overwhelmed, and are frustrated they aren't making progress. They're almost always thinking in the micro and missing the macro.

Jim Hart, an OTA student in Philadelphia, Pennsylvania, registered for the course after 25 years working with clients in person. Soon after, he emailed with a plethora of pressing micro decisions. From a name for his business, to enabling notifications in Google Drive, Jim was bogged down by the little things, finishing his email asking, "What do you suggest? Can I still be successful as an online trainer?"

Micro decisions add up, and Jim got to the point of questioning his path. But Jim simply needed to see that all of his micro stressors came down to the macros of fear and forgetting what matters most to clients: investing your time, energy, and money into providing the highest-quality service. After a couple back-and-forth emails, Jim was back on track.

Are we saying ignore the micros? No. They do add up. But in general, your clients won't care about them. So fix what needs to be fixed, but don't give micros any more time than they deserve (if you've ever worked for a micromanager, you know what it's like to die a workday death of a thousand micro cuts;* why do that to yourself?).

If any component of your training is causing you and/or your clients regular headaches, it's worth spending the time to shop around and switch things up. But beware trying to find the mysterious "best" what-have-you or geeking out on some program presentation that won't matter in the slightest to your clients. That way lies madness.**

The 10-10-10 rule is one of the simplest and most effective methods for "unsticking" your brain and moving you forward. This concept was first created by business journalist and author Suzy Welch, and is used across many industries.

So let's say you're dealing with any of the issues we've been talking about. You're taking too long with a choice

* The Chinese term "lingchi" translates to "slow process" or "lingering death" and is more popularly known as "death by a thousand cuts." It was a form of torture and execution in China from around 900 to 1905, when it was banned.

** A friend of mine is a world-class expert in developing learning models. He wanted to learn how to play guitar. Naturally, he set out to build a model for how to do it best. Six months later, he realized he had yet to pick up a guitar and strum a single cord. In his words, "If I had walked to the closest music store, bought the cheapest guitar, and googled a free guitar tutorial, I'd be six months ahead of where I am right now."

and you know it. Time for some perspective. First, identify the worst-case scenario that could result from taking action (this could range from "not much" to "I'll lose my business," so be honest with yourself). Then, ask three questions:

1. How will I feel about it 10 minutes from now?
2. How about 10 months from now?
3. How about 10 years from now?

Your answers will help you realize whatever's weighing you down probably isn't as life-changing as you think.

On the flip side, think of the *best* possible outcome and ask yourself the same three questions. You'll notice many of the stressors delaying you have a disproportionately high reward relative to risk when you take action, but you talk yourself into a corner anyway. Speaking of which...

When you talk to yourself, watch your language.
Perception matters. You want people to perceive you in a positive way, of course, but how do *you* think about you?

David Sarwer, a psychologist and clinical director at the University of Pennsylvania's Center for Weight and Eating Disorders, uses perception as part of his treatment. He gives new patients a mirror and instructs them to use gentler language when talking about their bodies. For sustained, long-term results, it's not enough for the weight to be simply lost or gained, but for the patients to morph their body perceptions.

How you perceive yourself and your business will determine how you act, even down to your day-to-day routine.

How can you use this to your advantage? Self-talk. Yeah, yeah, it's easy to laugh off or store in the category of "I don't need it." Maybe so, but its power and impact can't be ignored.

- Avoid negative self-talk.
    - "He's better looking."
    - "I'll never have as many clients as she does."
    - "I'm scared of failing."
    - "It didn't work for me but it's not my fault."
- Practice positive self-talk.
    - "My hard work is paying off."
    - "That person has a business I want. Time to learn from the best."
    - "I'm not afraid of success."
    - "I'm confident in my abilities. My clients wouldn't keep coming back otherwise."

Ever heard of Aesop's fable about the fox and the grape? A fox sees a grape on a vine that he can't reach. Instead of finding ways to bogart the grape, the fox tells himself the grapes are probably sour and not worth his time.

The lesson? *People belittle that which they think is beyond their reach.* As a result, we convince ourselves we don't want it.

It's easy to want something, try to get it, and, when it seems out of your reach, justify to yourself it's not what you want because it's too damn hard. Offer yourself some choice (positive) words and resist doing that.

Ask: Am I failing because of my method, or my approach? What is true in life is true in online training: A lot of different methods work. The missing element is often not the method, but a lack of patience, consistency, and implementation.

Some of our graduates see success in days, others months. Unfortunately, some give up before they see the rewards. What they don't see is the progress they're making. Instead of recognizing that going from a three out of 10 to a five out of 10 is progress, they compare themselves to others who began at eight out of 10. They get disenchanted, blaming themselves or, sometimes, "the system."

Check out this graphic (adapted from *The Fundamentals of Online Training*, the OTA textbook). So many people walk this path, seeing very slow upward progress. That can be frustrating because it looks like nothing's happening. But you've lit a fuse that's running beneath the surface of the positive things you do. The key is not giving up before the real acceleration starts.

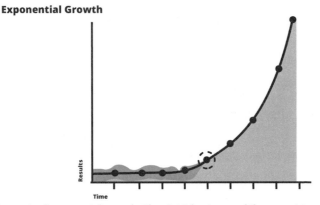

Exponential Growth

The magic of exponential growth: Slow initial gains — while not exciting — can add up to explosive growth later on.

News flash: You will fail. One day you may publish a status update asking for support and get no response, or a prospect will turn you down on a sales call, or something else. These failures are inevitable. How you respond will dictate your success.

Never forget that N=1 is not a reliable study. One person or one try is not enough to form a solid conclusion. You can't discredit anything unless you have sufficient data — and one, or a few, attempts is not sufficient data.

Choose a method that feels good to you and trust it, but never forget about your approach. Whether you decide to learn from us or somebody else, odds are that what they teach you will work, but only if you go at it the right way.

Ask: What would this look like if it were easy?
Maybe that sounds glib, but asking that question is one of the founding drivers of the OTA and it works. And it goes right back to the first sentence of this chapter.

When in doubt, simplify, simplify, simplify.

THE TAKEAWAY

New online trainers face decisions big and small. Understand the difference between choices your clients will care about and those that seem bigger than they really are. Focus on a positive mindset, hit your freedom number, slam-dunk amazing client service, and you'll do just fine.

CHAPTER 4

Identify Your Ideal Client

"The beauty of the internet is there's a niche market for everything, and if you can focus on it, you can build a sustainable and viable business."

—Michelle Phan

If this book has any goal, it's taking what we've learned at the OTA guiding thousands of trainers through their online transitions and helping you avoid mistakes (and we've seen 'em all). One place we see the most screwups? Client recruitment.

Who do you want to work with? Who's your ideal client?

Sure, every marketing and business book walks you through the "ideal client avatar" process, but even if you've deemed this step irrelevant in your head ("I'll work with anyone!", "I already know who my clients are!") let's put some more thought into it. Why? You're starting a new business. Online is not in-person. Which means online clients don't necessarily have to be the same type as your in-person clients (though they can be). You have choices. Possibilities.

Why pass that up?

Another reason: The more you read here and the further you get into your online business, the more you'll realize how fluid all of this really is. Strive for better, without question, but forget about "perfect." Perfect's a rumor. It doesn't exist.

That goes for every aspect of your new business, especially clientele. What you think you know today could change. In fact, most successful online coaches have tweaked their target audience since starting. They got out there, had some preconceived ideas, fumbled around, talked to people, and slowly figured out the types they wanted to train. Then they coupled that evolving info with their personal strengths and weaknesses to find their niche.

Let's start the process for you right here.

Welcome to the world of infinite shelf space

Before online coaching, almost every client acquisition

looked something like this:

Client wants fitness. *You're a trainer.* Client walks into gym. *You're there.* Client says, "I want training." *You say okay.*

Before online coaching, if a client in Beaverton, Oregon, wanted a trainer, she had the trainers in Beaverton to choose from — and likely just the trainers on her end of town (most clients refuse to travel more than 20 minutes to a gym).

Now a client in Beaverton, Oregon can work with an online trainer in Topeka, Kansas or Bangkok, Thailand. Location is no longer a factor and a person five miles away doesn't have to seek you out just because you're local.

The internet has given us a world of infinite shelf space, a phrase that grew out of, as you might guess, Amazon's dominance. Back in the day, the 'Zon started as an online bookstore. Compare its selection and prices to those at even the biggest Barnes & Noble store and there was no contest. Why? B&N had limited brick-and-mortar shelf space. Amazon had infinite digital shelf space and could offer any book title on the planet (now it's the same for toilet paper, portable air compressors, and fish oil).*

---

* *In his book* The Long Tail, Wired *editor-in-chief Chris Anderson shows just how much opportunity there is for everybody with infinite shelf space. In the "long tail" model, a few win out very big, but there's so much market opportunity that millions of smaller businesses can win over time, too. There's enough for everybody. It's very exciting!*

Online training made the same transformation. Now that anyone can hire any online trainer on the planet, we've eliminated "availability bias," which kept people working with coaches close by even if someone farther away was the better choice.

It used to be the same in a lot of other industries. You bought whatever brand of product your local supermarket stocked. You had just a few options of coffee to choose from, for example.

Not anymore. Now you can order any coffee you like online. Even niche companies can reach customers on the other side of the globe. The resulting effect is a decentralized, democratized, and open marketplace.

This means you may need to change your priorities. This means separating yourself in areas like niche selection and putting your uniqueness front and center. That's why identifying your ideal clients within a given niche is a big deal.

Online training is open and unregulated. This is good for you because it's easier than ever to enter the market. Unfortunately, if it's easy for you, it's easy for everybody else as well. Anybody can post shirtless pics on Instagram and call himself an online trainer. Guess what? You don't need to worry about those people.

The people who last in this business, the ones who stoke their careers and build businesses over time and love helping people, find ways to set themselves apart. They make it easy for potential clients to see why they're the obvious choice. *That's* why this online environment is so exciting. A wide-open market lets you set yourself apart. The single greatest marketing advantage you have, and will always have, is that there is only one of you.

This isn't about accumulating thousands of followers. It's about appealing to a faithful audience that trusts you and sees you as an expert, *their* expert. In any open marketplace, the best will always thrive because, in a market devoid of availability bias, the customer becomes the boss, choosing based on relationships, reputation, trust, and who she believes can best serve her.

This decision is rarely based on actual merit. Instead, it's based on an uncommon commonality that often has nothing to do with fitness. A great example: OTA student Troy Bennett, who has made himself the go-to fitness professional in the Chicagoland cosplay* community. The result? His first five clients signed up with no hard-selling necessary — all because Troy connected with them in their world (read his story here: **onlinetrainer.com/troy**).

Part of this conversation is marketing, and we'll cover that later. Right now let's talk about that boss customer...

---

* Cosplay is short for costume play. It's a growing trend where people dress in costumes representing various characters, usually superheroes or video game icons.

Who do you *want* to train?

This is the first step we see missed time and time again by trainers trying to find their niche. Who do you enjoy training? What ignites your fire?* What gets you out of bed in the morning? Enjoying what you do day in and day out is a necessary piece to the puzzle. Never overlook it.

Consider this story of an OTA student trying to find her niche: She offered coaching to her audience without specifying who it was for (she wasn't sure at the time) and 12 people signed up. Awesome, right?

Then she took a moment to look over her group. She noticed 11 of them were middle-aged women. Hmm. Not only middle-aged women, but women in similar positions in life, facing similar battles, and with similar goals. With some guidance from our coaches, she realized this was an attractive and valuable niche for her and hasn't looked back.

Is this how it will go for you? Maybe, maybe not. Don't dedicate your energy to worrying about that. Dedicate your energy to understanding yourself and your audience. Do that, and decisions tend to become obvious.

Find your blue ocean

Let's say you decide to be casual or vague with your

---

* Shameless, I know. Ignite the Fire *is the title of my first book:* **theptdc.com/ignite.**

target audience. Even good trainers make this mistake. What happens? You wind up competing with a plethora of trainers vying for attention, all getting frustrated that nobody is listening or willing to pay anything more than bargain-basement rates.

Some people can absolutely succeed without targeting. That success usually boils down to developing a network of trusted people from a variety of backgrounds, or maybe they have the secret sauce of good looks, charisma, writing/video skills, and luck. And I'm not dumping on that. If you're in a position to make that happen, get out there and do some good. But for most of us, in order to create an advantage, we need to go deep, not wide, to differentiate ourselves.

For example, let's say the bulk of your in-person clients were 20- to 60-year-old men and women who wanted to lose weight. It makes sense to use that mold for your online clients, right? The short answer: With a strong network you communicate with regularly, you'll likely get clients in this broad group (which is too big to be called a niche). But you'll fight for them in a red ocean* when you should be seeking open waters.

Create your blue ocean by differentiating yourself. Create a category of one and you'll become the obvious choice for your ideal client in an online marketplace.

That metaphor comes from Blue Ocean Strategy *by professors W. Chan Kim and Renée Mauborgne, one of the most notable business books in the past 20 years. It describes the process of developing "uncontested market space" — the blue ocean — while the rest of the competition tear each other apart for the same customers in a bloody red ocean.*

They'll find you, ask to train with you, and pay whatever you ask. Ignore this principle and you'll be just like all the other online trainers told by clients that your services are "too expensive" — and that's if you ever get a chance to talk to them.

Showcase your uniqueness

In the words of my friend, John Romaniello, the *New York Times* bestselling author and founder of Roman Fitness Systems: "What customers or readers react to and how they decide what to invest in is not based on the 99 percent of what we have in common, but the one percent that makes us different."

Clients don't choose you because you're like every other trainer ("I'll help you lose weight! Burn fat! Gain muscle!"). They choose you because of the one percent that makes you different. This is your 1% Uniqueness Factor.

Conventional is boring and gets ignored. Uniqueness sets you apart. Not a single other human on this planet is you, or has your perfect recipe of qualities and experiences.

That, friends, is a competitive advantage. Your uniqueness will attract like-minded clients, and because you've mapped this out, gone that extra step to set yourself apart, you assure those clients that you understand them on a deeper level than just sets and reps.

It also gives you a talking point when you contact the client. Think about it: When you reach out to a potential lead, would you rather say, "Thanks for your query. My prices for training are XX to YY. Would you like to get started?" Or would you prefer to say, "Wow! You love Indiana Jones, too. Did you know Spielberg cast Tom Selleck first? Think he would've been as good as Harrison?"

Finally, it helps you pick out the people you really want to work with. Your time is your most valuable commodity. Asking questions to predetermine whether you'd enjoy working with a client is just as important as learning their exercise histories.

> *Going two inches wide and two miles deep when seeking clients will always serve you better than the opposite.*

Example: OTA student Michael Sotos, from Ashland, Oregon, lets his uniqueness and generosity shine when clients join up at Uncanny Strength and Conditioning. Michael's application, which is meant to appeal to superhero fans, has fields such as "Special Abilities and Powers" and he also asks applicants to name their favorite superheroes.

Why? For one, it shows a sense of humor and that training with him won't be deadly serious. Two, it creates a connection with others who share a similar interest, and is more likely to move the needle for that population. And three, Michael sends clients a figurine of their favorite superhero along with a note thanking them for purchasing his services.

Brilliant. This is just one example, but Michael was able to take something he already enjoyed and use it to build a deeper connection with his clients. You can, too.

How do you appeal to your niche?

To connect with your niche in a personal way, you can also tap into shared experiences. Other trainers who haven't gone through the same experience simply won't "get it," even if they can empathize.

Some examples:

- An army veteran working with other military personnel.
- A new mom training other new moms.
- A trainer who used to be obese, who understands that journey, working with other people in a similar position.

Now, does this mean that a male trainer who wants to work with new moms shouldn't do it? Of course not. But it's a simple fact that a new mom will have an easier time marketing to new moms because she can tell her story.

Ideally, your clients should feel like they "get" you. They should feel special that they recognize something in you because you reach them on common ground.

Meet clients where they are

For you literal-minded folks, we don't mean where clients are standing right this second. Like, at the coffee shop. Though you can try. We won't stop you. No, this is a basic concept about connecting with them on an emotional level.

Remember, the easier you make it for a client, the better chance he'll sign up. So let's look at ways trainers make it more difficult to connect. We'll start with the most powerful tool you have: language.

The right language can bridge a gap; the wrong language can make it wider. Case in point: Trainers love to use trainer language. Words like "performance," "mobility," and "hypertrophy" are everyday parlance for fitness pros. But the general population? Eh, not so much. Sure, some people will respond to jargon. But in an ideal world, you want potential clients to think you're speaking directly to them. It's personal.

Making your prospects learn a new language becomes just another barrier standing in their way. If you don't already have their trust and attention, that's not a mountain you want to climb. A really good example of "clients vs. jargon" is Weight Watchers. They produce lots of magazine and online articles to help their

members with fitness, but they avoid using the terms
"exercise" and "workout" in the copy.

Sounds crazy, right? A weight-loss company avoiding
the most common fitness terms? Not really. Here's
why: About a third of WW's members are "normal"
exercisers who run, bike, or go to gyms. Another third
walk, and that's about it. The other third don't exercise.
The mission of WW's content is to engage *all* members,
so they strive not to unintentionally intimidate or
judge the folks who don't exercise. They use terms like
"movement" or "physical activity," which have nothing
to do with gyms or formal exercise, but just might
inspire non-workout folks to get moving.

When thinking about language, put yourself in your
clients' shoes. How would *they* describe the benefits of
your services? What problem(s) are they attempting to
solve, in their words?

A perfect example is Carolina Belmares, an OTA
graduate and owner of Sweatglow Fitness. Carolina
charges substantially more than anyone in her town,
both for in-person and online training. Her ideal clients
are affluent, and to get to know them better — and to
show them she cares — she attends the fundraising
events her clients support.* When she does, her clients
go out of their way to introduce her to others and she
gains easy referrals. Not only that, by schmoozing with
lots of her ideal clients, she learns the language they
use, their unique challenges, their frustrations, and

---

* *Okay, so you can literally meet your clients where they are.*

their goals and limitations. Her empathy, as a result, is genuine.

If you don't have immediate access to a live audience like Carolina, find mass-market authorities who serve your audience and analyze how they communicate and connect. This can be in:

- Advertisements
- Books and magazines
- Videos
- Websites
- Social media profiles

How do they reach prospects? How do they define problems? How do they sell solutions? While you don't want to copy or steal their words, you want to communicate to your audience where they are in a way that triggers a reaction. This process can pull back the curtain.

Another way to whet your appetite for this type of work is to find other companies and coaches who promote to your target population. Buy their books, subscribe to their emails, follow their social media feeds, and be a sponge. Pay attention to the language they use and, in particular, what gets a good response and what doesn't. From here, you can take what is useful, adapt it into your own unique offering, and leave the rest behind.

"CAN I TRAIN PEOPLE OUTSIDE MY NICHE?"

Coach Alex here. I get that question at the OTA all the time. The short answer: Of course you can. Just because someone doesn't immediately identify with your niche doesn't mean you can't click with them in a trainer-client capacity. This is particularly true when you're just starting out and need clients.

Think of it this way: Your niche gives you direction. It helps dictate where you invest your time and efforts and guides your communication. It's the shovel you're going to use to carve out your own corner in this industry.

That said, building a network of people who know, like, and trust you takes time. Opening yourself up to your current network where that trust is already built-in is a great way to get your first few clients.

How do you appeal to your existing network while being clear about what you do and who you help? One strategy is to remove the specificity around the demographic you train, while maintaining the specificity around how you help them.

Take this niche as an example:

"I simplify fitness for busy female entrepreneurs ages 25 to 45 and help strengthen their bodies and minds through flexible online coaching that they can fit into their hectic schedules."

That's a pretty good niche. Still, while building up your foundation, you can expand your reach with a simple shift:

"I simplify fitness for busy people and help strengthen their bodies and minds through flexible online coaching that they can fit into their hectic schedules."

This isn't a permanent solution, but it's a great way to cast a wider net getting started and begin getting some momentum. Remember: Niche or not, as long as you get along with your clients and they respond to your direction, you'll get results.

Ah, but here's the thing: *You* may not like the words you find in these environments. You may know those words don't actually mean anything, or that they're not being used correctly, but you need to work through that. Meet clients where they are, not where you wish they'd go.

Some trainers might say, "Wow, that really isn't me. That's not how I want to operate." Going against what you believe can be tough. You need to decide what you're okay with. For instance, some trainers would loathe using words like "toned" or "functional" or "lose belly fat." And that's completely fine. Know that about yourself. But also understand that your audience likely possess different perceptions about that language, and you may be creating a barrier by not meeting them where they are.

There's more: Many fit pros live in the online communities of other professionals and we take pride in the approval of our peers. When you use language that resonates with your prospects, you may get pushback from other trainers. That's completely okay, too.

Remember who you've set out to help. Remember whose business depends on reaching clients on a gut level.

Proceed accordingly.

THE TAKEAWAY

If you identify your ideal client, you make it easier for the two of you to find each other. You'll share similar interests and goals, and if you develop your niche, you'll have clear access to potential clients in that niche. The more common ground you share, the happier everyone will be.

CHAPTER 5

Pricing and Packaging Your Services

"Always render more and better service than is expected of you, no matter what your task may be."

—Og Mandino

We're talkin' money again, and yeah, it always messes with people's brains. How much should you charge for your services? How should you package those services? What, after everything is said and done, are your talents really worth? Good questions. That's why there seems to be this mysticism around pricing in the fitness industry.

Some pros are terrified of charging too much. Others are worried they're charging too little. *Where's the sweet spot and how do I hit it?*

Understand: It ain't magic, or some secret recipe, or
something to be scared of. Pricing, however, does have
power. It represents your vision and dictates your
actions. And it can communicate more about your
business to a customer than any other marketing piece
or headline you can create.

If you respect that power and learn how to harness it,
you'll eventually arrive at price points that will satisfy
you *and* your clients. Here's how...

The psychological power of price

Think about your gut reaction when you see a price
tag.* If it's cheap, you think it's low quality. If it's
expensive, you think it's high quality and more valuable.
Does that always turn out to be true? Of course not.
But we're talking about instant psychological reactions
here. Be honest: You're slightly intrigued when
something seems outrageously expensive, aren't you?

You see where I'm going, but I'm not advising you to
price yourself outrageously high just for the sake of
pricing yourself outrageously high. Still, think about
what happens when a customer shops around for
trainers and comes across two options with one that's
double the price of the other.

---

* Caveat: We don't mean a piece of expensive merch marked down to
bargain levels. This is a fully priced hypothetical example.

The immediate reaction: "Hmm, that trainer's a lot more expensive but looks really good across the board." Now, whether the customer chooses to pay is a different discussion. Some customers will always choose the cheapest option, but you don't want to work with them anyway. Let other trainers appeal to those bargain-basement shoppers.

Also, charging twice as much means you need to work with half as many clients to make the same amount of money. That opens you up to more professional development, more side projects to generate income, develop your business, or spend more time with your family or on a hobby or working out.

I personally shudder at the idea of working more hours for less money. Don't you?

Find the right price for you

There's no ideal price point for online fit pros. The "right" price is simply what works for you.

A lot of newer trainers will "shop around" looking at what other trainers charge and base their pricing on that. Beware the compare game. No two trainers are alike. You're complicating something that should be simplified. Agonizing over something you had the answer to all along.

I won't walk you through a magic pricing process. That would be pointless. Rather, I'd like to share a few principles and strategies. The magic will come from you. Why? You'll develop your pricing from your own business structure and what kind of business you want to run, not from what other trainers are doing. (Yes, it's true, celebrity trainers like Chris Powell can sell programs for much cheaper than you can. He can also sell *a lot* more, and appeals to a completely different audience than you. If you do desire to sell thousands of programs, you'll need to do the work that no one sees, spending years — if not decades — building your brand, networking, and achieving mastery to get to where Chris is now.)

Rather than worrying what everyone around you is doing, look at:

- Your freedom number.

- The value of your time.

- The services you offer and the time it takes to create and deliver them.

- A realistic assessment of the hours you want to work, keeping in mind you also need time to grow, develop new ideas, and market.

All of those things will be unique to you. No other trainer will have identical answers to yours. That's why you need to be careful when looking at what other pros charge. You can, however, look at how other trainers work through this process. Once done and at your freedom number, you can then decide whether you want to expand and scale. Some do, others decide that they are happy where they are. The choice is yours, and that's the point.

For example, a recent OTA graduate named Sara took the time to determine her price objectively. Based on what she wanted to offer her clients and how much time she had, Sara needed to charge $800 a month, and could only take on four clients at a time.[*]

Her response: "I could never charge that much! It's too high. Nobody will sign up."

We talked about her situation. The numbers didn't lie. Sara is a qualified life coach and wanted to include a substantial amount of private coaching calls with her package. While powerful, these calls take a lot of time and increase what she needed to charge. She had to decide what to do with the objective truth in front of her. She had two options: The first was to remove some of the more time-consuming aspects of her service to lower what she needed to charge. The other was to accept the situation as-is and find four people who would pay $800 a month.

I mentioned that pricing represents your vision and

To find this number, she used the Online Training Pricing Calculator that we provide within the Online Trainer Academy. It takes into account freedom number, services, how much time a trainer has to deliver her service, and how long her desired package will take to deliver, then provides a variety of pricing options at different client quantities. Our coaches then guide students like Sara to their ideal business structure. This, of course, is prone to change over time, which is why many of our students return to this exercise multiple times over many years (students have lifetime access to both the Online Trainer Academy materials and our coaches at no extra or ongoing cost).

dictates your actions. Sara's story is a great example. She had a vision and once she knew what she had to charge, her required actions became clear: She needed to go after affluent clientele, which affected everything from her sales voice to her marketing channels. Sara went from "I could never charge that much" to knowing that, for what she wanted to deliver and how much time she had to deliver it (she's a busy mom), she *had* to charge $800. It didn't take long for her to integrate herself into more affluent communities, rebrand her materials to give them a more prestigious feel, and take on the four clients she needed.

And with only four clients, she did an incredible job and gave them an exemplary service, which made generating referrals easy. Sara now has the perfect turnkey business for her, in her time, generating enough income for her family *without* taking away her time and attention. That's the power of precise pricing.

The pitfalls of higher price points

You need to grasp an important concept: *If the right kind of prospect understands the value in what you offer, price becomes increasingly irrelevant. On the flip side, if a prospect doesn't understand the value in what you offer, or isn't the right person for your services, any price will be too high.*

If a client decides that you're the person to help them become the version of themselves they want to become, that's priceless. A prospect in this frame of mind won't bat an eye at practically any price you present. However, a prospect still thinking *Why should I work with this person?* will question practically any price you suggest.

Another important point: *No matter how low you price your services, there will always be clients who cannot afford you.* Even if you do all the right things and make a killer sales presentation, some clients will still say you're too expensive.

When they do, you'll be tempted to drop your price. And why not? Fitness businesses can grow fast by driving price as low as possible and stealing members away from other clubs or fit pros. Isn't that the name of the game?

No. Don't fall for it. When low price is your only advantage, it's just a matter of time before a competitor undercuts you with even lower prices. The market quickly becomes a race to the bottom, squeezing profit margins to razor-thin levels and eventually driving everybody out of business.

This pattern has run its course multiple times in the past few decades, and surely will again. You don't want to be in a fight like that. The only winners are extremely large and efficient businesses and, even for them, the margins are so thin that the smallest change in market conditions can take them out.

"Wait a second," you say. "All this flies in the face of logic." The best product at the best price will always get the sale, right? This couldn't be further from the truth — and leads to a lot of frustration from people in the fitness industry who believe they know more and are better professionals than the ones who have taken the time to learn marketing and, as a result, build bigger businesses that help more people.

It's time for you to start paying more attention to your price, figure out the pricing model that works best for you, understand what you're unconsciously communicating to your clients with that price, and adjust your marketing accordingly.

What should you offer for that price?

Beware the temptation of offering too much. That's the mark of an *un*confident trainer. Always err on the side of underpromising and overdelivering. This is a good way to go for a couple reasons:

First, you don't want to overwhelm yourself, and that's easy to do. Just because you're working online doesn't mean you're working smarter. I've known quite a few trainers who didn't put enough thought into their packages and ended up working twice as hard for half the money online.

Second, clients who do well with a remote trainer are self-motivated. It's not your job to be there every second, performing endless phone check-ins* and over-assessing. Your job is to provide clients with the support, direction, and accountability that they need. You'll empower and encourage them so they can take ownership of their fitness — and enjoy the process.

As trainers, both in-person and online, it's commonplace to discount the time we spend preparing for clients, offering support, and doing our own administration. The "pay for service" model of training where we earn an hourly rate is likely the culprit.

If you're going to have more freedom in your personal and professional life, you need to break free of this mindset. You must appreciate the time it *actually* takes you to deliver a service in order to value it. You may be surprised what you come up with.

Here, I'll list out a whole bunch of potential services you could include in your packages. I recommend that you estimate the amount of time it will take you to deliver that service *before* you consider offering it.

TEMPLATES: THE SHORTCUT TO EXCELLENT PROGRAM RESULTS

The more ways you can find to save yourself time without compromising customer service,

---

* *Nobody needs to speak to a trainer every week, or even every two weeks. And phone check-ins should be just that, check-ins lasting no more than 10 to 15 minutes. Have a list of quick questions to run through to give you an idea of where your client is with training and recovery.*

the easier your job will be — which allows you to focus more time on your business and clients (a virtuous circle if there ever was one).

Templates save you time and prevent you from building a program from scratch for every new client.

I understand you may think templating strips away individualization of each program, and thus does a disservice to your clients. Nope. If you do templates correctly, the opposite is true.

The fact is, most clients can be bunched into categories. The workouts for all clients within a single category will be similar. That's where templates come in. Meanwhile, as you work with a client over time and take in more feedback from them, you'll continue to individualize and iterate on the initial template that you provided.

That's the trick: Templates should serve as the foundation of each program that you individualize as you develop a deeper understanding of your clients' goals and desires.

Create a basic template for every client goal, such as hypertrophy, mobility, fat loss, and strength.

What likely won't change from client to client:

Programming considerations. *Things like sets, reps, rest, and tempo will likely stay constant.*

Order of exercise categories. *While your first exercise may not always be a bench press, it's likely to be some sort of multijoint, upper-body horizontal push for similar clients.*

Workout split over the week. *How many times the client trains and how the programs are split over the course of the week likely won't change much.*

What likely will *change from client to client:*

Specific exercises. *While the exercise category will stay the same, the specific exercise may change.*

Grips, implements, and stances. *Physical limitations, previous injuries, and access to equipment will vary by client.*

Possible service ideas

This list is not exhaustive. There are always other ideas. I don't suggest that you offer all of them (that would be crazy). This is a chance to consider your options and what may work best for you and your clients, as that's always the most important piece.

- **Custom program design.** All the individualized workouts a client needs (sort of anti-templating).

- **Custom nutrition design.** This may take the form of a meal plan and/or nutritional guidelines.

- **Daily tips.** Sent automatically through your email system, these could include health and habit tips delivered daily or at regular intervals.

- **Phone consultations.** Weekly, biweekly, or monthly phone consults, ranging from 15 minutes to an hour.

- **Email / instant message support.** Answering program questions, having clients send you pictures of their food, or responding to general concerns may apply here.

- **Guided movement screen.** Initial movement assessment over Skype, in addition to regular check-ins.

- **Assessments of any kind.** You could include anything from strength tests to endurance tests to body fat measurements.

- **Membership program.** Access to a password-protected platform that delivers tips, hosts a community, and provides additional support.

- **Positive messages / affirmations.** Simple but powerful motivators. May include pictures, quotes, or personal notes.

- **Mindset training / life coaching.** For those trained in these types of coaching, you may include them as part of a full transformation program.

When it's time to put your packages together, I recommend keeping things simple and starting with two offerings: one that includes little-to-no support and one that requires more of your time.

Here's an example of two potential core packages:

1. Custom workout program design + initial video assessment + biweekly 15-minute phone call check-ins.
2. Custom workout program design + custom nutrition design + initial video assessments + monthly video assessments + biweekly 15-minute phone call check-ins + weekly email support.

The difference between these two packages is how much personal support you provide. Your basic offering delivers some core services with minimal ongoing support. The second, more upscale package offers extra personal care.

A FUN WAY TO GENERATE BUZZ

Along with all the services you can offer, think about trying a competition. A contest or something similar can bring your business positive attention while showing a lot of people how you can help them achieve their goals. The trick: Now your clients are competing with each other (and themselves) for the best transformation.

A good contest/competition should include the following pieces:

Two deadlines: One for clients to register, and one for members to hit the predetermined goal.

One specific goal that appeals to one audience and can be achieved in a short period of time.

A fun name that lets people know it's for them, and when the contest is happening. For example, "Summer Slimdown!" is concise and catchy, but more important, it tells your audience that this is a contest for people who want to firm up for swimsuit season.

A clear method of determining the winner.

Cool prizes! Cash, gift cards, spa treatments, workout apparel, and more. (Pro tip: Local companies or online retailers might want to work with you to provide prizes in exchange for promotion.)

The easiest way to get a contest off the ground is tying it to a season or holiday. To start, pick a holiday or event that is at least four to six weeks from the start of your contest. So, "Summer Slimdown" may start in the middle of April. Your

> *contest doesn't need to correlate with a season*
> *or event, and could just represent a goal of your*
> *members. "Tighter Tush" anyone?**

The key for you: Consider all the nuts and bolts of what you'll have to do to make your services a reality. Understand the time required not only to get the service up and running, but to maintain it. If you don't have this very basic understanding, you're going to have big problems later on.

Let's look at Online Trainer Academy grad Gina Patterson from Bend, Oregon, as an example. Her nutrition and training business, Bite Nutrition, offers the following services:

- Accountability and support
- Training tips
- Meal planning strategies
- Training logs
- Custom nutrition plan
- Custom training plan
- Initial setup call
- Detailed reviews
- Email support
- Private check-in calls

---

* *Alliteration for the win!*

All of the above is offered in her low-end package, however only a nutrition *or* training plan is provided. Her high-end package includes a custom nutrition *and* training program, in addition to all of the services offered in her low-end package, and it's as simple as that.

Of course, Gina's just one example. Let's look at another one.

OTA grad Ren Jones from Charlotte, North Carolina, and owner of Fitness Jones Training, offers three packages: basic, premium, and executive. His basic package includes:

- Live initial movement screen assessment.

- Customized training program.

- Biweekly phone check-ins

Ren's premium package not only increases the frequency of his phone check-ins to weekly, it includes customized nutrition coaching, sleep coaching, and guidance around injury prevention and recovery.

The executive package ramps up his support and offers two weekly phone check-ins, daily text message motivation, as well as two 30-minute face-to-face video calls each month. He also tacks on a one-year nutrition program in addition to separate monthly "no equipment workouts" for road warriors.

The bottom line: There's no magic formula of services to offer. It all depends on who you help, what problems they want to solve, and what fits with you and your expertise. Don't worry too much about what others are offering. Dedicate that energy to figuring out what makes the most sense for you.

THE TAKEAWAY

Don't undersell your services. Build the business you aspire to build and price yourself accordingly. People generally associate higher prices with higher value. Charge what you believe you're worth, exceed those expectations every day, and clients will sign up.

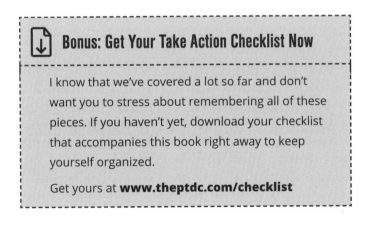

Bonus: Get Your Take Action Checklist Now

I know that we've covered a lot so far and don't want you to stress about remembering all of these pieces. If you haven't yet, download your checklist that accompanies this book right away to keep yourself organized.

Get yours at **www.theptdc.com/checklist**

CHAPTER 6

Client Onboarding and Physical Assessment

"A stunning first impression was not the same
thing as love at first sight. But surely it was an
invitation to consider the matter."
—Lois McMaster Bujold

Some folks have a real talent for making other people feel important. That's the kind of talent you need to develop if you want to become a successful online fit pro. I'm talking, of course, about your clients. Results are the priority, but if you can make them feel important, valued, and respected along the way, they'll never leave you.

That starts on day one. When you sign up a client, what happens? What do they get from you? What do they see? How do they feel? How do you *make* them feel?

Welcoming new clients — a.k.a. onboarding — is the first experience they'll have with you aside from any previous sales process. In other words, this is your client's first impression of how you operate. Onboarding will kick off your professional relationship on a good, awkward, or not-so-good note.

Onboarding is also a critical opportunity to further appeal to your niche, separate yourself from the pack, strengthen your relationships, and continue to cement your personal brand and reputation.

Oh, and proper onboarding is good for one other thing: Identifying and potentially weeding out clients who won't click with you or your program. That sounds negative, but trust me, it's a positive. Client-trainer mismatches help no one.

So let's look at some onboarding basics, including how to perform an effective baseline physical assessment online (that is, from a distance).

Your application form

A potential client is interested — so much so that she's about to start your online application form. What will she see? And what information do you want from her? This is your first transaction with her. What needs to happen in the next few minutes to ensure that (a) she buys in and (b) you have a really good idea of what kind of client she'll be?

You see, the application is not a one-sided process. It's not just, "Oh, plug in your name, email, and credit card number and we're good to go." You *and* the client have a stake. Your form is another source of information that'll help you underpromise and overdeliver. It's also an opportunity to cement the relationship.

Your application form has three main purposes:

1. Build rapport.
2. Gather pertinent information.
3. Qualify leads (i.e., determine if that client is a good match).

So what questions should you ask? Keep it simple and let your personality drive the tone. Some trainers are all business. Some keep it light and fun. Any tone is fine as long as it's honest and reflects your practice, because you'll attract more like-minded clients, and those who aren't a good match won't click (literally and figuratively). Some application strategies to keep in mind:

–   Collect the basics: Name, age, weight, gender, email address, etc. Sounds obvious, but little things are easy to forget.

–   Ask about physical limitations, medical conditions, injury history, or special considerations when it comes to workouts. This isn't just for your information. Conditions could tie in to the client's goals ("I want to get off my diabetes meds!") and state of mind ("I get so angry when I look at the scale!").

- Use questions that hint at what's to come in the trainer-client relationship, but also let you know what kind of client that person may have been in the past. *What's your fitness goal? What kind of workouts have you done previously? Have you worked with a trainer before? How open are you to trying new things?*

- Use questions to your advantage. You should not only include fun and creative questions that showcase your personality and build rapport, but also try to weed out clients you don't want to work with. This could mean asking potential clients to rank their commitment level, or if they're willing to invest money in improving their health and fitness.

To help qualify the leads that come her way, Online Trainer Academy graduate Michelle Rycroft of Ripped by Rycroft includes the following questions on her application form:

Are you willing and able to invest $40 per week into getting the results you want?

How committed are you to losing stubborn body fat?

She also does a great job building rapport with questions like, *What's your favorite gelato flavor?* But including those first two questions identifies people who aren't a good match before they get too far.

Meanwhile, OTA grad Lee Kinghan of Phoenix Nutrition and Fitness helps qualify leads with this final question in his application form:

Do you understand that no magic pill, wrap, juice cleanse, or tea will get you where you need to be, and that hard work is ahead?

That's a mic drop right there. Those who don't align with that approach won't apply, and those who do, will. And that's the goal with qualifying questions like these. Don't be concerned that some people won't want to train with you. It's more important to attract clients who will be the right fit.

AMA ABOUT FAQ

Your online headquarters should definitely have an FAQ section and you can even encourage potential clients to "ask me anything." Enthusiasm for answering questions hints at patience, honesty, and transparency. That'll give people one more reason to like and trust you.

When you receive a question about your program or services, add it to a running list of questions and answers you have on hand. This can be posted on your website, as well as sent in each client's welcome package. This keeps your FAQ

> *consistently growing and up to date. And yes, if
> one person asks about something, chances are
> someone else will wonder the same thing. FAQs
> are a great vehicle for offering information about
> you and your business.*

Your welcome package

If your application is a chance to offer a great first impression, your welcome package is a chance to blow people's doors off. Make it your hard-and-fast rule: Each new client gets a personalized welcome package immediately after signing up. Remember, you're working with folks remotely, so your package will ideally be digital (you certainly could ship a physical welcome package with similar swag you'd gift to a new gym client, but that gets unwieldy over long distances).

An effective welcome package brings two things:

Fun: Welcome clients to your training and get them excited. Reinforce why they chose to train with you.

Facts: All the information they'll need about how the online training process works and how to work with you.

Here are some examples of what you could include. You don't need to include everything on this list, and this list is not exhaustive by any means:

- *Thank you and welcome.* This can take many forms.
  A quick note, a full letter, whatever feels right.
  You can do the straightforward route, or create
  something visual, or make people laugh. It's really
  up to you. Just make it a genuine reflection of you
  and your business.

- *Introduction to the program.* Clearly define it,
  including why it's so effective. Speak directly to
  your clients. Emphasize how your program will
  benefit them.

- *Procedures for working with you.* This is crucial, for
  this part helps manage client expectations and lays
  out the rules on how much interaction you'll have.
  Texting and email have spoiled us* in a way, because
  they're so immediate and convenient. But trust me,
  you want strict guidelines for how often a client can
  contact you. Here's what I suggest:

- The client can send you one email a week.

- The email must be all bullet points.

- Each bullet point is a question or comment.

- Each bullet point can be a maximum of three
  sentences.

---

* *My friend Andy Morgan, owner of RippedBody.com, an online training company operating out of Tokyo, Japan, has a "no cellphone rule." When a new client registers, they sign off that they will never contact him via cellphone. Over sushi when I was visiting Tokyo, Andy told me that no intelligent message was ever sent via a cellphone. I don't know if I'd go that far, but I certainly agree that forcing a client to only contact you by computer weeds out a high percentage of wasteful, thoughtless messaging.*

- There can be an unlimited amount of bullet points.

- A client can send you the email at any point of the week, but you'll respond to it at a predetermined time each week (you determine this and stick to it).*

Of course, with this structure built into your program, you can still make exceptions. You can always be a human being first, no matter what guidelines you have in place.

If a client is struggling, go ahead and have an extra phone call, or offer additional support. The important part is to set expectations around your availability so that you don't feel pressured to offer 24/7 support. If you make an exception for a special circumstance, your clients will appreciate that you are going above and beyond.

Watch your language, redux. When clients get an online training program, it's likely the first time they've seen a personal trainer structure services this way. It's important to make that structure simple and clear. Someone with no fitness background should be able to look at your services and understand exactly what they will be receiving, and exactly how they will benefit.

---

* Consider the impact of these simple, yet eloquent, rules. If left to their own devices, people will fire off questions without thinking, write in long and redundant blocks of words, and ask way more than what's needed. By putting these rules in place, you still offer unlimited support but create an ecosystem in which they write succinctly, organize it for you, and only ask what's necessary.

Remember: The language you use is important and can either bridge or widen the gap between you and potential clients. Speak their language. What's common to us can be foreign to our clients.

I learned this the hard way when I first started training. After demonstrating a dumbbell overhead press for a client, I got all enthusiastic and said, "Okay, let's do three sets of eight and see how we feel. Ready?"

I was met with a blank stare. "Wait, three sets of eight?" she asked.

"Oh, sorry," I said. "Three sets of eight reps each set."

Still looking confused, she asked, "What's a rep?"

Hey, it happens. One way to add some fun to any potential language barriers is creating a "Handy Guide to Trainers' Jargon, Lingo, and Nonsense" with a collection of definitions and "translations to English" (or whatever language is appropriate). Again, fun *and* facts.

- *FAQ* (as previously discussed).

- *Links.* Maybe you have a video library, or have published on blogs or in magazines. The videos will be especially important if they'll help clients understand program elements.

- *How physical assessments will work* (more on this in a minute).

- *Common mistakes.* 'Cuz you just never know.

- *Gym etiquette.* Always a worthwhile education since good gym etiquette is so rare and makes the world a better place.

- *A guide to workout recovery.*

- *A sample workout from the program.* Include instructions on navigating the software you use, if any.

- *Cancellation/refund policy.* Keep it simple and transparent.

Again, these are just starting points. This all comes down to understanding your audience. For example, OTA student Ruvi Makuni of Fit Active Toned includes most of the basic information listed above in her welcome package. But she also adds an extra few pages on how to keep yourself accountable, guidelines on getting a good night's sleep, and helpful advice to differentiate between good pain and bad pain.

Why do all that? Ruvi primarily works with busy professionals, and she not only understands not only how important safety, accountability, and sleep are to her clients' progress, but also that those things are the first to go south within that population. So she makes sure her clients never overlook them.*

Ultimately, your welcome package should give clients all the info they need to succeed. Remember: It's your clients' first peek behind the curtain. They just invested in you. Don't take it lightly. Allow empathy to guide

---

* *Want an example of a great welcome package? Check out the PDF Ruvi sends to new clients here:* **onlinetrainer.com/ruvi-welcome.**

much of your decision-making here. Put yourself in your clients' shoes and visualize their experience. How would *you* like to be welcomed to a new program? What would make *you* feel valued and important? Do likewise.

And now a few words about fine print

Unfortunately, every business requires some amount of fine print, a.k.a. legal language that protects you and your clients. Hear that? That sound was all the fun being sucked out of the room. Yes, it's tedious and can be intimidating but there are certain legal pieces that every online coach should have in place.

We'll cover some fundamentals in this section, but understand there are simply too many differences from region to region, country to country, to get specific with the details of legal or liability issues. The safest and most effective way to ensure you're fully covered and meeting the requirements of your jurisdiction is to consult a local attorney. It's worth the investment.

What will you need? Client signatures on these basics: a liability waiver, terms of service, and a privacy policy. In addition, you'll want professional liability insurance that covers online clientele.

Let's look a little deeper into each of these pieces:[*]

---

[*] *Online Trainer Academy students get these three forms built for them through a proprietary generator included in the digital portal that takes in each trainer's personal information and creates the necessary documentation.*

- **Liability waiver.** This document communicates the potential risks of the service you offer and ensures the client will not hold you accountable should an injury occur while working with you.

- **Terms of service.** A set of regulations that your clients agree to before they begin working with you. This will typically outline your policies and procedures around payments, cancellations/terminations, intellectual property rights, and more.

- **Privacy policy.** How you'll gather, use, disclose, and manage client data. This includes any personal and payment information.

You can include these documents in your welcome package. You can either have clients print, sign, scan, and send them back to you, or integrate your documents with a platform where clients can "sign" digitally.

Liability insurance

Insurance for online training* should cover you in two scenarios:

1. The client has never seen you in person.
2. The client can be located anywhere in the world.

Often insurance will cover online training only if you have seen the client in person before, or if she lives in

* *The Online Trainer Academy has gathered a network of worldwide insurance providers that meet the criteria above for our students.*

the same insured region as you. If these scenarios meet your business setup, you're good. But if not, you'll need to adjust your coverage.

Your certifying body will likely partner with an insurance provider. And while it's not guaranteed that this particular provider will meet your requirements, it is a great place to start your search.

How to do a baseline physical assessment online

You may have heard the medical expression that doctors shouldn't "diagnose from a distance," meaning they should never make a judgment call on a patient's condition without seeing the patient in person. That doesn't necessarily apply to personal trainers doing an initial physical assessment of a new client, but if you're training someone online and "from a distance," you should adjust your approach.

Before we begin, let's clear up a misconception. Assessing clients online without being physically present is absolutely possible, most of the time. As we discussed in chapter one, some clients shouldn't be trained online at all, and these clients shouldn't be assessed online either:

- Clients in any sort of rehabilitative process.
- High-performance athletes.
- Clients who have never exercised before.

For everybody else, remember an assessment has two purposes:

1. Develop a physical baseline to work from.
2. Identify any major limitations/injuries to refer out to a medical professional when necessary.

The big difference between in-person and online: **Online assessments must favor reliability over validity.**

Most coaches have been trained to favor validity with assessments and, for reasons that go beyond the scope of this book (in other words, long story), the test-to-test reliability of many assessments commonly done in a gym is low.

I'm not downplaying the importance of having valid measurements. It's always better if you can get them, but the reality is most tests aren't valid anyway. Take body fat tests, for example. Unless your client has access to DEXA, Bod Pods, or underwater weighing, any test result they've been made to believe is valid just isn't.

It's even harder to get precise, valid measurements remotely and I don't suggest you try. Why? You can get reliable information from basic assessment protocols that are easy for your client to do at home with little guidance (meaning they're hard to screw up).

The following are some common assessments that work well for online trainers because they're reliable. Keep in mind that different types of clients will need different assessments, so you'll want a few options in your arsenal. And if you have a different method that works for you, great. Keep using it.

—*Body fat.* This is the most common assessment. We all know body fat is better to measure than weight. Unfortunately, it's also more difficult and requires measurements with calculations, or in-home devices that are notoriously finicky. And those body fat scales are basically useless.* As popular as body fat is, I suggest...

—*Tape measurements.* Tape measurements are a good, old-fashioned method and you can find free online calculators to estimate body fat from those numbers. A tape measure is cheap, and since an inch is an inch is an inch (and a centimeter is a centimeter), measurements are reliable. You'll have to coach a client on how to use a tape and trust that they are reporting honestly.

—*Body weight.* Your biggest problem won't be getting clients on the scale; it'll be getting them off it. Clients tend to care too much about what the scale says and

---

* Most gyms use a form of bioelectrical impedance to measure body fat. This is commonly done with scales but can also be performed using electrodes hooked up to a person's body. The machine sends a current through the body and measures resistance, which gives an indication of body fat. The problem is that hydration, which can be affected by everything from liquid consumption to sleep, varies and adds an element of error from three to five percent, rendering the test more or less useless. As researcher James Krieger says, body fat testing with bioelectrical impedance is a prediction, not a measurement. If you're interested in more of the science, Krieger has published a great four-part series on his blog Weightology that you can find here: **weightology.net/bodyfat.**

weigh themselves far too often. Like many trainers, I don't like tracking body weight, but it's so culturally ingrained and so easy to track you almost can't avoid it. Because of that, the OTA suggests advising your clients to only step on a scale once every two weeks.*

What should you care about from a progress standpoint? Tracking weight once a month to note improvements and set new goals is a good general rule. Also, remember that a client may have positive progress without losing weight, such as adding muscle over fat where they feel or see physical progress even if the number on the scale doesn't budge.

—*Movement screens.* Functional Movement Screen (FMS), individual screens, or assessments of specific movements (such as a squat or walk-back-and-forth) can be assessed through video, either live or recorded. Movement screens are generally performed over Skype (or a similar video conferencing service) where you can cue the client. Alternatively, more advanced clients can record themselves based on your instructions.

—*Max lifts or 3RMs.* A max lift should only be requested from an advanced lifter. It's now commonplace for those who coach powerlifting online. The average client won't need it.

—*Fitness tests.* Old-school tests — 60-second push-up or

---

* Since you and I both know your clients will weigh themselves daily despite what you say, have them track their weight using an app like Happy Scale (IOS) or Libra (Android). These free apps smooth out the curve showing overall progress and not the day-to-day fluctuations that can be hard to swallow for some clients.

crunch tests, shuttle runs, flexed arm hang, etc. — can be surprisingly useful in online training. While the tests won't tell you that much in terms of absolute fitness, they form a great baseline and show progress well. Another benefit of this type of assessment: It creates a distinct goal for a client to surpass, celebrate, and talk about.

—*Endurance tests*. Most often, cardiovascular tests are given to athletes as a way of measuring everything from efficiency to strength to improvements in work capacity. If you work with an athlete, you'll want to adapt the test to the specific demands of their sport. For general population clients, a good old-fashioned beep test, one mile, or 12-minute runs work well.

Basically, you're going back to gym class.

Ready to rock and roll

If you take this chapter in chronological order, from signing up a client to sending your welcome package to performing a baseline physical assessment, your end result should be a coach and client who are prepped and psyched to start training. Through all of this, your clients should feel like they're about to get into something big. Exciting. Life-altering. Because they are. And they should be just as pumped to have you as their one-and-only guide.

THE TAKEAWAY

Client onboarding done right simultaneously gets your new clients even more excited and lets them know the ground rules of your online relationship. Your onboarding process should reflect your personality and program, establish expectations, and make a client feel valued and important. Think of the entire process as a launching pad for a great working relationship.

CHAPTER 7

How to Deliver Online Training

"When you can do a common thing in an uncommon way, you will command the attention of the world."

—George Washington Carver

It doesn't occur to many trainers that launching an online business component can be incredibly creative. As in, if you open your mind to new ways to run things or solve problems, you'll find unexpected fixes that can be cheaper and easier than the "expected" ones.

Case in point: It may surprise you to know that you don't have to pay for software to run an online training business. Which sounds crazy. After all, "online" implies that coaching software isn't just optimal, but necessary. Nope. In fact, many trainers use their own concoction of free services like email, Google Sheets, and Google Docs (or paid software like Microsoft Office) to formulate a system that works for them and their clients.

But hey, maybe you want specific software that's an all-in-one solution and makes your life a zillion times easier.* We'll talk about that. Just remember: None of the following suggestions are commandments. Like with everything so far in this book, the important piece here is developing a system that saves you time and mental energy.

Let's take a look at the three most common ways online trainers deliver their services:

Old school

Some folks are hooked on anything "old school." That's fine. Old school here means using readily available software applications to trade information. Here's how it works:

1. Using a spreadsheet program like Microsoft Excel,** write all of your client's programs manually into a template. Include instructions or videos for how to perform some or all of the exercises.
2. Email the program to the client.
3. With no way to track progress on a regular basis, you'll have to follow up constantly to ensure the

---

Approximately.

*** Lots of great, and free, workout templates are available online. I like the ones offered at **exrx.net/WeightTraining/Instructions.***

client is working out and ask for updated data. (For example, if he weighs and measures himself on a weekly basis.)

4. Once the program is finished, you'll need to get complete data. Ideally, clients will be filling out a workout tracking sheet (date of workouts including weights, sets, reps, etc.). They could scan or take a picture of a workout they've just completed.

5. You'll need to input the data into your own system and chart it to identify trends, usually on a master spreadsheet.

6. Once a client completes the program, you'll have to repeat the process with a new program, updating your existing data on this client.

If this sounds like your worst nightmare, you're not alone. Yes, it's cheap, but it's also labor intensive and requires disciplined computer time. Imagine doing this with 20 clients. I don't recommend it. Of course, if you know this is the route for you, do it the best way you can. But you have other options...

Cloud-based

Pretty straightforward here: Use an internet-based (i.e., cloud-based) storage drive to operate your business, giving clients access to a shared folder where they can download and upload files as instructed.

For simplicity (remember that?), we'll talk about Google Drive, a cloud-based storage solution available to anybody who has a Gmail account.* Google Drive is great because you can create documents within it and share permissions to either view or edit with whomever you like. It's also free and easy for anyone to use.

Google Drive offers a free program called Google Sheets, a simpler version of Microsoft Excel, which allows you to easily produce templates for your workouts.

You might be quick to point out that working within Google Drive is similar in some ways to the old-school model. True, but with one major difference: clients upload their own data into a folder you've created for them. All you need to do is create a folder for each client and share permission so you both have anytime-anywhere access.

Anytime-anywhere is the key. The client can access workout sheets on a phone or computer when he's ready and fill it out (at home, at a gym, in a hotel room, 24/7 anywhere he can get online). Meanwhile, you can monitor his workouts in real time.

This process is about as good as it gets without paying for software.

Yeah, let's talk about that...

---

* As of this writing, Google Drive is ubiquitous and we couldn't possibly imagine a world without it. But times change fast in the tech world, so you may be rolling your eyes right now and wondering why we're not talking about "Next Disruptive Supercompany's Cool Stuff." Hey, the platform may shift but the advice is still timeless.

Software

Every day, in one form or another, we're asked, "What's the best online training software?"

> *If you need a deep dive into specific training software, the Personal Trainer Development Center now has a completely updated software resource that analyzes options. Check it out here:* **theptdc.com/software.**

Not much has changed since we spoke about this in chapter three. As with every decision you make, don't strive to find the "best" option. It doesn't exist. There's only what's best for you and your clients. If you're able to make your business work for you so you don't have to worry about technology, you'll have more time to dedicate to helping clients solve their problems.

It really is that simple: Instead of spinning your wheels trying to find the capital-B best, use the time to figure out your own needs. Good training software allows you either more free time or the ability to take on more clients. As a result, software you pay for should be a good investment. Most OTA students begin without software and adopt it later after taking on their first few clients.

THE TAKEAWAY

Delivery options for online training range from free cloud-based services to pricier software designed just for trainers. The key: Forget what everyone else is doing. Find the method that serves you and your clients best. That's the criteria for any decision here.

CHAPTER 8

Client Retention, Feedback, and Testimonials

"The customer's perception is your reality."

—Kate Zabriskie

Your job is keeping clients around.

"Wait, what? I thought my job was training clients? Getting them results, remember?"

The great results, the fantastic customer service, the enjoyable rapport — those are tools for getting the job done. And the job is keeping clients around. Look at it this way: It's a lot cheaper in time, effort, *and* money to keep an existing client than it is to find a new one. Getting clients on board is one thing, keeping them around is another, and it's the latter that will ultimately determine your long-term success in this field. And the longer they stick around, the better their results will be.

There are a lot of ways to do that, from very basic to very creative, and we'll get into them here. We'll also get into feedback and testimonials, which reflect client satisfaction and also help shape your brand.

The first step...

Make your clients feel like all-stars

Clients come for the training, buy for the people, and stay for the relationships.* Think about the people you share a deep connection with in your life. Do you feel this way toward them because they did one thing that stands out? Or because they did a lot of the littlest, imperceptibly caring things over a long period of time?

PUT RENEWALS ON AUTOPILOT

Part of client retention is renewals, and your online training business should have a built-in process for that. A simple strategy is autobilling that renews clients for a predetermined package, paid either biweekly or monthly.

Any online merchant system, including PayPal, allows you to set this up with a few clicks. You can create a few different subscription buttons programmed to charge regular amounts at

---

* Write that one down and hang it on your fridge.

> *whatever intervals you set up. You can create one*
> *system for everyone or a unique payment link for*
> *each client.*
>
> *And if a client wants to stop training with you?*
> *Cancel away.*

While there isn't just one thing that I can single out for you to do, I will help you identify a number of those impactful little things that you can do for your clients, day to day, to cultivate a bond that transcends a mere client-trainer relationship.

It's not complicated. It's also not automatic. It's not something you can optimize, or check off a box when you're done. You have to be purposeful day in, day out, essentially making your clients the center of your universe. They have to feel important because, let's face it, they are.

The power of strategic gifting

Unfortunately, most trainers (heck, most people) stink at giving gifts. If it's the thought that counts, well, it's obvious that very little thought goes into most gifts. Holiday and birthday cards? Meh. A bottle of wine? Forgotten the morning after it's drained.*

A creative, thoughtful, unexpected gift can be your advantage. If you've spent some time finding the

---

* *Depending on the severity of the hangover.*

perfect little thing for a client, they'll remember. Again, it's not complicated, but it's not automatic, either. To make it easier, run every gift you give through this filter:

- **Is it personal and personalized?** The best gifts mean something special to each person. The cost of the gift is insignificant. This shows you know your clients, listen to them, and value who they are.

- **Is it disposable?** The best gifts can be used over and over again. Think about gifts in marketing terms. Typically, you might measure a marketing effort in something called cost per impression (CPI), and if you think of your gift in terms of CPI, your goal would be to maximize the number of impressions per dollar spent on marketing. A bottle of wine will be used once for a single impression. Not really worth it in those terms. But personalized wine glasses for a wine lover could be used endlessly and the client remembers your gift with each sip.

- **Is it expected?** Sending a holiday or birthday card each year is nice, and appreciated, but it creates expectation. That elevates your risk while diminishing your reward. One missed holiday or birthday and whoops, people notice. The best gifts come unexpectedly at random times. This is how you separate yourself from the crowd.

- **Is it top of class?** More expensive doesn't matter, but top of class does. A $25 personalized porcelain coffee mug is a better gift than a $100 watch. Why?

Because the coffee mug will be the best mug that they own and they'll use it every day. The watch, on the other hand, will be low quality or a substandard brand for that much money.

BECOME A WORLD-RENOWNED GIFT GIVER EVEN WHEN $$$ IS TIGHT

If you're just starting your online business, money may be tight and gifts cost money. Not big money, but the expense can add up if you have multiple clients. Consider terrific gifts you can give that cost you nothing but a little time and bandwidth. Example: Shoot a video celebrating a client's new PR or other milestone and send it when they least expect it. It'll have the same value to the client even if it didn't cost you a dime.

Here's a great example: OTA graduate Alisandra Khairuddin[*] of FitNut Loft went above and beyond for a client's 100th session. Aly surprised her with a bound book of her journey, customized with the colors she normally wears to work out, and embossed with a personalized note on the front. The icing: Not only was the client floored by the gift, she didn't know she'd hit

---

* *In Alisandra's own words, "I was a Precision Nutrition Client and loved their curriculum and software, so I jumped at the chance to use it (loved being PN certified, too). But, then what? How do I get my name out there? I got these answers from OTA." Read her story here: **online-trainer.com/alisandra.***

such an amazing milestone and was filled with pride.

"She was so damn proud of herself," says Aly. "I was so proud of her. And the other ladies in the class hugged her and cheered her on. Thinking about a gift made such a huge difference, rather than giving a free class or socks."

This is the power of strategic gifting, and what surprising and delighting your clients is all about.

Another example: OTA grad Amber Bonem of Glow Mama Fitness has an older client who loves softball and still plays. Amber attended one of his games to show support, took action shots of him playing, and used them to create eight custom trading cards personalized to him.

Brilliant. That's a gift he'll never get rid of or forget, and it was offered for no good reason. That's how you do it.˙

Make accountability fun

Accountability will likely be a primary reason clients sign up with you. They know what they have to do to achieve their goals, they just need some confidence, consistency, and encouragement to execute. That's part of a trainer's job. The problem? Keeping accountability positive but not heavy-handed.

———————————

** Want more great gift ideas? Go to **onlinetrainer.com/gifts** for more examples of remarkable gifts sent by our students that cost less than $30.*

One easy way to do this: Celebrate your clients every chance you get. Use small wins to highlight progress. How you celebrate is up to you but it needs to be fun, effective, and personal. Some ideas:

—*Mail your client a certificate and stickers*. Every time they train, tell them to put a sticker on the certificate. (And no, they don't have to be gold stars. But who doesn't like a gold star?)

—*Set up (or automate) check-ins*. Have your client send you a photo of every meal eaten or a post-workout selfie. Send them a thumbs-up emoji in response. Even simpler, messages like, "Hey, on a scale of one to five, how was the workout today?" or "Hey, just wanted to check in. One to 10, how did you sleep last night?" can make an impression.

—*Send a note*. Unexpected handwritten notes of encouragement are a cut above texts and emails.

—*Use an app*. Encourage your clients to use a fitness tracker or habit app, not because you care about the data but because it allows them to see results and celebrate the process.

—*Use software*. If a client uses training software to log completed workouts, the process of filling it in and seeing a completed workout is an opportunity to celebrate.

ANATOMY OF A GREAT CLIENT CHECK-IN

In the accountability bullet points, you'll notice I gave scales to these check-in notes (one to five, one to 10, and so on). The point of a short check-in is creating a constant line of communication that doesn't require a lot of thought or drawn out conversations. You're checking in to show you care and get wind of issues before they become problems (sleep quality, for example, is a big indicator for recovery and stress).

Our students use a variety of methods for check-ins, from email to FB/IG messenger to text message. Some of them also opt for an automated text message service like Off Day Trainer which sends out texts from your number on a schedule (i.e., one a day at random times) and the response goes to you. This is just one example of using technology and automation to scale your ability to make personal connections and coach better on an individual basis.

For our Online Trainer Academy students, we have prewritten and loaded up the Off Day Trainer system with 50 messages, or for those students who don't want to pay for this software (or don't live in the USA — the only place it's

available, unfortunately), we provide all 50
messages on a spreadsheet and they can send
them out manually, once a day or every few days.

Client spotlights

As long as you have permission, showcase your clients
and their stories to your audience. Keep it short, bring
the awesome, and make it all about the client with the
following:

- Images (such as a before-and-after, or just a regular
  photo).

- A few words about what they did to make the
  change.

- Any hardship or struggles.

- A motivational, excited, and congratulatory finish.

OTA grad Thomas Madden of Satellite Fitness does
a fantastic job showcasing not only his clients'
achievements and the obstacles they've overcome, but
also their varied backgrounds (women, men, young,
old), increasing the chances that someone reading will
think, "This could be me."

Most important, he emphasizes what the results mean
to each client. They did all the work and that should be
celebrated. Then Thomas leaves a link to his application
so anyone who's curious can take the next step.

In Thomas' words: "As challenging as one might think

the OTA is, it's the ABC's of creating a great business
— which is exactly what I needed. There's no filler,
no BS, just straightforward actionable steps. Also,
what company has this kind of support? It's like if
you were having enough trouble, a coach will get on
a plane and come help you figure stuff out. I am no
longer on an island by myself. Now I have a tribe. I
have support, guidance, and a clear path toward a real
live business. My biggest complaint is that whenever
I would implement something, I'd get new clients,
which slowed me down a bit." Read Thomas' story here:
onlinetrainer.com/thomas.

Encourage client feedback

A client feedback system is two things: A no-brainer
and a win-win (or is that three things?). Go all Nike
and just do it. Receiving feedback is a great way for you
to hear how you've been doing, what you could be doing
better, and ultimately how to keep your clients coming
back. It's also an effective way to gather testimonials.
Asking for feedback shows your clients you care enough
to not only listen to them, but make adjustments based
on what they say.

The simplest way to implement this? Make it an integral
part of the program. When clients sign up, make sure
they know you ask *all* clients to fill out a feedback form
(or customer review, or whatever you prefer to call
it) every two to three months because it helps you
constantly improve. You can automate these intervals

through an email system, or use calendar alerts to remind yourself to reach out.

Let's talk about effective strategies for getting and using client feedback...

Stop asking clients for testimonials

Testimonials are an important tool for any online trainer. Not only are they a great way to showcase what you do and who you help, but they can play a major role in your client acquisition. The problem? Getting them can be, well, icky.

While clients may write something nice about you if you ask them to, they also may not get back to you. Following up can be awkward. You also can only ask for a testimonial once, maybe twice, over your training life cycle with a client.

The solution: Stop asking for testimonials. Instead, incorporate a process of systematic reviews of your training into your program (as mentioned, every two to three months works well). If you're doing a great job, a customer review will automatically become a testimonial.

To engage clients (and not waste too much of their time), a simple online survey is quick and efficient, and will collect vital info if you ask the right questions.

Ah yes, the questions. What to ask? Honestly, there are a million different questions you could ask on these surveys in a million different variations ("How awesome am I?" is not one of them), but let's make it simple for your clients' collective sanity.

Ask three questions.

Only three? Yup, that's it. I've found the following three questions, taken directly from Scott Stratten's excellent book *Unmarketing*, provide more than enough information:

1. "What's one thing you want me to keep doing?"
2. "What's one thing you want me to stop doing?"
3. "What's one thing you want me to start doing?"

See? Very simple and straightforward. That said, you don't have to use these questions. Feel free to come up with your own, and use more than three, especially if you have very specific questions you're dying to ask. The key is respecting your client's time. Five minutes is reasonable, but 10 starts pushing it.

A sample script for the first message you send out for feedback:

"Hey (Name),

This is a quick note to ask for your help. It should only take five to 10 minutes of your time today or tomorrow.

I'm constantly working to make my online training services better and it'd mean the world to me if you provided some feedback.

Attached here is a review form. On this there are X questions, some specific to us working together and others to help me learn more about you.

Thank you in advance for your time. Not only will this survey help me get better, but it will help me serve you better in the future too.

—(Your Name)

A sample script for every time that follows:

"Hey (Name),

Well, it's review time again. It should only take five to 10 minutes of your time today or tomorrow.

Like I said a few months back, I'm constantly working to make my online training services better and it'd mean the world to me if you provided me some feedback.

Attached here is a review form. Some questions are specific to us working together and others will help me learn more about you.

Thank you in advance for taking the time. Not only will it help me get better, but it'll help me serve you better in the future too.

—(Your Name)

You can send your form as an attached Word document that they fill out, scan, and send back, but the best way is to create a Google Forms survey one time, and give your clients the link.* This way all responses from all clients will be neatly organized in one place.

Important note: Be sure to include a checkbox giving you (or your company) permission to use all information in this form for any marketing and/or promotional efforts in the future. If someone checks "no," you cannot use it (and it would be horrible if you did).

From there, you can do one of two things:

1. Use what they wrote verbatim.
2. Massage what they wrote into a single text-based testimonial. If you do this, it's a good idea to send the statement back to your client for approval, even if you already have permission to use it. Be respectful. A simple, "Hey (name). I'm so happy you're thrilled with the training so far. I've taken the liberty of rewriting your review into a sort of testimonial for my services. It's copied below. Do I have your permission to use it in marketing and promotion moving forward?" works fine.

The before-and-after photo: a classic

Before-and-after-photos are a powerful promotional

---

* *There's a ton of free web forms you can use. Google Forms are great, but I totally get it if you're (not-so) secretly terrified of the all-mighty Google. Other options include Wufoo and Typeform. They all work fine.*

tool and a great way for a client to showcase aesthetic progress. The easiest way to generate these photos is to ask for them as part of your training program (and be sure to secure permission before you use any photos).

HINTS FOR A GREAT BEFORE OR AFTER PHOTO

—Use the same pose and take the photo in the same place to make ongoing physical changes stand out.

—Get three angles: front, side, and back.

—The area should be well-lit.

—A white backdrop works best.

Some software programs make it easier by enabling clients to take the photo with their phones directly within the app. The photo is then date-stamped and uploaded to the user account for you to check.

Now all you have to do is showcase the photos — ideally combined with a testimonial — on your website or social media feeds. And there's the win-win: Clients are happy to show off their incredible progress (and keep training with you), you're happy to show off your coaching skills (and maybe recruit new clients to boot). Everyone's happy.

THE TAKEAWAY

No matter how well you coach, get results, or connect with clients, if you can't retain them you won't have a business. Use personalized gifts, feedback, testimonials, and celebrations to make your clients feel like all-stars. Their loyalty is everything.

CHAPTER 9

Four Foolproof Marketing Strategies for Online Coaching

"Our job is to connect to people, to interact with them in a way that leaves them better than we found them, more able to get where they'd like to go."

—Seth Godin

You've come a long way. You've laid the foundation of your online training business and now it's time to take another step: marketing your program.

Marketing for trainers could be many books all by

itself.* For our purposes here, let's dig into four simple but powerful marketing strategies you can implement immediately. You won't need a big ol' marketing budget or any formal marketing knowledge or experience. All you need is what you've already brought to this book: A desire to work, learn, try new things, and improve.

Let's start at the beginning...

#1: Sell to people who are ready to buy *now*

Here we'll cover two very basic marketing tools that require minimal resources and yet can deliver good results. And as that headline states, you should be positioned to convert the easiest candidates because, hey, they're ready to sign on *today*. All you need to do is connect.

—*Build a website.* You're running an online business, so having a state-of-the-internet website is the first step, right? Well, not really, no. It sounds counterintuitive — a web-based business without a web presence? — but it's true. Building a website is not necessary to be a successful online coach. In fact, for most folks just making the transition, I'd wager a website is near the bottom of the priority list.

Now, I'm not saying it's useless or a waste of time. I'm simply saying it's another tool at your disposal. That

---

* In fact, we've gathered more than 200,000 words of leading-edge business advice from the most successful names in the fitness industry in Fitness Marketing Monthly: The Complete Collection. *If a marketing master class for fit pros exists, this is it. Check it out at* **theptdc.com/fmm.**

said, keeping this tool clean and sharp can certainly play to your advantage and be an effective way to sign those who are ready to work with you. It can help strengthen your brand, showcase your services and personality, and ultimately help you build a network of stronger relationships.

There are literally hundreds of ways to build a website. And you're a beginner. You know what that means: Beginners complicate, experts simplify. It's waaaay too easy to get wrapped in the minutiae of building the perfect site.

Take a breath and be realistic. One of the biggest mistakes you can make is putting a huge amount of time toward your website before you have any clients. That's a form of procrastination. Good enough is fine, especially at the start. Get something up that accomplishes the basics, then move forward. You can always make improvements later.

The basics:

- **Home page.** The job of the home page is to let users know they're in the right place and invite them to explore.

- **About page.** The about page should build rapport and connect with the website visitor as a person. A high-quality photo accompanied with a brief introduction from you is a good start. Of course, it's crucial that this entire page is *not* about you. Do the brief introduction, but transition into why you got into training your niche and how you help clients solve their problems. Pro tip: Use more "You's" than "I's" on this page.

- **Services page.** Your potential clients likely don't trust you yet, so the goal of a services page is to turn visitors into leads, not to make sales. Instead, provide *just enough* information about your services and the benefits they bring. Then invite readers to learn more by connecting with you.

- **Contact page.** The contact page lets 'em find you. Oh, and people should feel welcome reaching out to you, not like they're intruding on your time. Provide complete details, including an address so people can associate you with a physical location, even if you work remotely.

Also consider two optional but helpful pages:

- **Success stories page.** We covered client celebrations, before/after, and testimonials. This is Celebration HQ, where visitors can see how you've helped people similar to them. Include any clients who have gone through fantastic transformations, or anyone you feel hits your niche well or can connect with people in your target audience.

- **Blog page.** A blog is a great tool to showcase your authority and provide value to your readers. Blogs don't have to be long essays. You can create how-to guides, tip sheets, personal stories, lists, and other forms of helpful resources. If the idea of writing blogs makes you want to crawl into a cave and never come out until the word "blog" has evaporated from human vocabulary, yes, you can skip it.

If you'd like to take a look at really good real-life websites of OTA students, we've linked to several here: **theptdc.com/online-training-websites.**

Despite everything written here, don't let website development delay your progress. If you don't have a site yet, register a free account at about.me and get a quick one-pager up. It's free and won't take you more than a couple of hours. Use that as your home base until you get your site together, and keep making forward progress.

—Capture those ready to make a change with this simple and effective script. My most common response to trainers telling me they have no idea how to get clients is, "Have you asked?"

You won't truly know how many clients are sitting in your network ready to make a change *today* unless you ask them. Here is a simple, succinct, and effective script to post to your audience on social media and via email.

I'm looking for five (type of person here, such as gender or age) who want to:

—Benefit X
—Benefit Y
—Benefit Z

Spots are extremely limited to five who are ready to make a change today. To apply, fill out the form and I'll be in touch if you meet the requirements:

(link to your application form)

Now here's an actual script created by trainer Mike Gorski, creator of MGFitLife.com:

Hey friends in the Madison area, after the awesome success of my 8-Week Strength Beach Body Group, I am starting a new advanced training 10-week group at Hybrid Athletic Club as soon as possible!

I'm looking for 3-4 more men or women looking to lean out, get strong, and build sexy bodies, that live in the Madison, WI area, who can work out at 6AM Monday, Wednesday, and Friday.

I am looking for people who want to:

- *Get stronger, and see how strong they can really be.*
- *Shred body fat and reveal muscle they never knew they had.*
- *Build confidence in yourself through a commitment to fitness.*

Spots are extremely limited and I'm only looking for 3-4 more people who are ready to make a change today. To apply, fill out the form below and I'll be in touch: (link to sign-up form)

If you'd like to explore this further, and also see how to create a sign-up form in Google Forms, check out

theptdc.com/new-client. As you go through this process, remember: The number of clients you're looking for can change, but it's important to be honest. If you're open to taking on 10 new clients and have 10 spots available, don't say you only have five.

#2: Become the obvious choice when people are ready to buy

This is a really big one. Without it, you'll struggle. With it, you can't miss. Software and good systems are important, but if nobody views you as an expert, no magical computer program or social media platform is going to help you.

All that matters is your reputation.

The good news? You have a lot of power at your fingertips. The fitness and health industry is one of the most profitable in the world. And you, as a fitness expert, are at the forefront. When you're able to establish trust and create a reputation that precedes you, you can sell in abundance and won't have a problem being paid what you're worth. But, like anything worth having, building this reputation takes time and, unfortunately, there seem to be a lot of impatient people looking for quick wins with surface-level techniques. Don't get frustrated. Do it right.

For people to trust you, they need to have heard of you. Blasting an advertisement in front of them, regardless of how persuasive it is, is not a long-term strategy.

Many of the tactics you see promoted heavily are fuel
for the fire and have their time and place, but you gotta
build the fire first. Here's how:

—*Carve out your category of one.* Take every word of
chapter four, "Identify Your Ideal Client," and apply it
again here. Cut through all the boring, expected layers
of yourself to get at your 1% Uniqueness Factor. Be
transparent, real, raw, and honest.

Our students tell us that the most common reason
why their customers buy is always something like "I
referenced an obscure Star Wars fact in an email"
and almost never because they talked about the
"Best Ways to Blast Belly Fat." Be weird, be wacky, be
unapologetically you.

But there's more: Use that uniqueness to position your
services in a way that makes you the obvious choice to
the right person, and the wrong choice to the wrong
person. Identify your position and confidently brand
it as yours, independent of what else is out there.
Own it. Commit all of your resources to dominating
this position. Avoid incestual marketing practices.
Refuse to be compared. If you think you're competing,
you've already lost. See, when it comes to selling
training, there is no "best," but winners control the
conversation.

How to do this? Try to bring new perspectives to the
table. You may work in a niche that feels familiar, but
what do *you* bring to it? What's *your* angle? Think of

some of your favorite movies. Whether you like action movies or romcoms, your favorites probably feel familiar to the genre, but the filmmakers found ways to give you something that was also satisfying and surprising. That's your goal: Give 'em something they haven't seen before, even if the niche sounds familiar.

Trust me, it's quite fun being the only game in town.

MY "1%" SOLUTION
BY ALEX CARTMILL

Hi, it's Coach Alex again. You may remember me from such memorable places as chapter one, "The Foundation of a Successful Online Trainer." Seriously, though, I manage a team of Online Trainer Academy coaches and mentors who interact daily with our thousands of students, and I wanted to share a story with you about how to set yourself apart.

When I remind OTA students not to shy away from their uniqueness, I ask them a simple question: Imagine a client is searching for an online trainer, and during their search, they find you and five other trainers who work in the same niche. "New moms," for example. Why should a client pick you when she's found five others who deliver fantastic programs for that population?

What makes you different, and how could you render price irrelevant?

This idea originally entered my life during the first conversation I had with Jonathan Goodman, a phone call to discuss a mentorship opportunity in 2014. After five minutes of back-and-forth, he asked, "What makes you better than trainers who are 20 years older who have 10 more years' experience?"

I didn't have an answer.

"As soon as you figure it out, let me know," Jon said.

I thought about it. Worked on it. And while my answer will be different from yours, I wanted to share the message I sent Jon on June 3, 2015:

Hey Jon, about a year ago when we spoke on the phone for the apprenticeship opportunity, you asked me what separated me from someone with 20 years' experience in the fitness industry. I had no idea. You told me you knew what it was, but I didn't. This past year I've been thinking about it daily, and it's really helped me shape my mindset and outlook on not only fitness, but how I live my life. I wanted to share what I've learned.

I thought things like my knowledge, work ethic, or communication skills would separate me, but I realized that's what everybody works on to separate themselves. It's important, but not enough. The first thing I learned is, the ability to articulate your passion goes a long way. When people noticed that I convinced some successful folks to write for free on a collaborative blog I ran, some wondered, "Who would do that?" They do it because I leave everything on the table. I tell them exactly what my vision is, what I admire about their work, and how I want to share their knowledge with others to make the world a better place, and it's blown my mind to see how many people are willing to come on board when you approach them with this attitude, as opposed to trying to sell them on something.

I also learned life is literally anything you want it to be. You have the ability to dictate your emotions, perspectives, everything. This was a mindset that was tough to make a habit; nothing controls how you feel or what you think, only you. Once I embraced this, I (1) became much happier, and (2) realized the amount of power a single person has and the impact he can have on others. This idea

fuels my fire and pushes me to take a ton
of risks and embrace failure, things I have
come to realize are vital to success as well.
This is the product of months and months
of thinking logically about what separates
me from someone with more knowledge and
experience, and it's helped me in business
and life. I just wanted to share that with you,
and thank you for planting that thought in my
head a year ago.

*This took me almost a year. I messaged Jon
knowing full well he'd forgotten about our
15-minute conversation 15 minutes after it
ended. I figured Jon liked my answer and that's
why he took me on as an apprentice. I later
learned that he didn't like, nor did he dislike,
my answer. What he liked was that I had taken
the time to think about it. That action, in Jon's
words, was proof that I was different and was
special. Jon doesn't look for people who know
everything. He looks for people who have taken
the time to think about who they are and what
they want because, in his words again, that's the
secret sauce and people who have it cannot fail.*

*That first lesson he taught me was to not rush
the process. It was almost a full year from when
we first spoke to when we worked together.*

Don't get me wrong, I was training clients and working the entire time, but the process cannot be rushed — and that's what I tell so many of the trainers I now mentor. If they can't come up with an answer in a few hours, they feel doomed for failure. Nope. It took me a year. So take a deep breath. You already have the answer. You just have to let it out.

#3: Provide value through content

When people talk about "networks," the first thing that comes to mind is probably social media. But your personal network that exists offline is far more valuable. In fact, more than 90 percent of word-of-mouth referrals still occur offline. This isn't talked about because it can't be measured but, as with so much else, what can't be measured is usually more valuable than anything that can.

Building your network is relatively simple. You say hello. You wish people well. You express genuine excitement around what others are doing. And you look to support others in their endeavors as much as possible.*

As you continue to build your network through genuine acts of generosity, share your journey and your knowledge. And yes, the majority of this will happen on

---

* A friend once told me to "never resist a generous impulse." This is some of the best business and life advice that I've ever gotten.

social media and via email newsletters.

A word to the wise: Don't try to do too much. Walt Disney once said, "Get a good idea and stay with it. Dog it, and work at it until it's done, and done right." Trying to do too much and be in too many places will not only exhaust you, it'll dilute your efforts. Instead, choose one platform and give it your focus and attention for a minimum of six months.

When thinking about a platform, don't overcomplicate it, but consider the following:

- Where will you find most of your existing network?

- Where do you spend most of your time on social?

- Which platform is best suited for your interests and skillset?

For example, if you know you like to write, YouTube is a bad choice. If you love video, YouTube is where you want to be. I refuse to give you concrete advice because that would be a disservice to you. What's "best" in the digital world is constantly changing and you don't necessarily need best because just about everything will work as long as you stick to it and build a community.

Once you choose a platform, as I said, spend a minimum of six months mastering it. Learn everything you can about it and ignore all else. Go deep, not wide. Not only will this tunnel-vision help keep you consistent, it'll allow you to develop a richer understanding of what your audience wants and needs.

Part of mastering a platform is understanding lead generation, networking, and content marketing from that platform. If you're trying to do a lot of things at once, you'll never be effective at any. Everything works, but only if you work at it.

After six months, you can decide whether to double down on your existing platform or expand into another one. Our best students almost always stick with what they're doing because they're having so much success.

#4: Ask and follow up. Then follow up some more.

If you want to get clients, you have to ask people to be your client. Profound, I know. Multiple times a week you need to share that you're accepting clients. The more specific way you ask, using the language and desired goals of your ideal client, the better success you'll have.

In our Facebook group, Online Trainers Unite, coaches post every day looking for advice on getting clients. The confounding part of it all is that, in almost all cases, they haven't yet asked their existing network if they want to train. *Ask.* Oftentimes it's as simple as that.

Then, after you ask and somebody shows interest, follow up. I've had experiences where I have pleasantly and politely followed up for three years once a month before a client decided to start training. In my experience, if you don't follow up multiple times, you'll miss out on at least 80 percent of your potential sales. Never be afraid to follow up.

None of these marketing methods are sexy, but they all work. I've decided to share them because the best methods are timely, yet timeless. I readily accept that at any given time there may be in-vogue client conversion methods that work for very short periods of time. In the Online Trainer Academy, we coach our students on these only after they've shown promise, but they never form the base of what you do.

The tried-and-tested methods are your foundation and, for most, the foundation is all you'll ever need because once you do an amazing job, referrals take over and do the heavy lifting. A lot of online trainers struggle long-term because they fall prey to one-and-done shiny-object tricks and techniques. Even if they work, which is a big "if," they won't work for long. The trainer then must reinvent themselves, looking for a new "best way to get clients." After a few cycles of this relentless and exhausting lead generation, they give up.

Marketing done right isn't fancy or complicated. It's simple and, just like building a great body, requires an obsessive, relentless, and consistent application of the basics, day in, day out.

THE TAKEAWAY

Some of the most effective marketing methods for fitness pros are the simplest: Building your online brand, setting yourself apart, networking within your niche, and following up.

CHAPTER 10

The Secret to Effortless Sales

"Sales are contingent on the attitudeof the
salesman, not the attitude of the prospect."
—W. Clement Stone

Before you start selling your online coaching, you need to understand what you're selling.

Sure, you're selling customizable programs, and maybe nutritional guidance, or accountability, or any other feature of your services. When thinking only in these terms, any amount of money is going to seem expensive if all you're selling is an online program, a flatter stomach, or bigger arms.

You're selling something much deeper than that, something much more valuable.

You're selling confidence. You're selling clients the

version of themselves they want to become. You're providing them the tools to create healthy habits that will last them the rest of their lives.

When you think of it that way, you're getting into the head of the person deciding whether or not to work with you. You need a deep understanding of where your clients are in their lives and where they want to be. And that's exactly how you should communicate the benefits of what you do. Sure, you help people "with their fitness," but you're also helping people live the lives they want to live.

Getting clients to recognize this value starts with *you* recognizing this value.

The most successful salespeople aren't always selling

We get questions on a daily basis in our free Facebook group, Online Trainers Unite, asking how to sell to clients. The question usually looks something like this: "I've tried everything. I have my website set up and I'm sending out Facebook ads and scripts and I can't get any clients. How are you guys getting clients?"

My response is always the same: "How many people have you spoken to today?"

Radio silence. Then, maybe a reply: "I've been posting

on social media and I've built 273 different funnels."*

To which I reply: "How many people have you spoken to today?"

And the answer is always zero.

So many people think sales is all about tactics like Facebook ads. Ad platforms have gotten easier to use, and as a result, more people are using them. This means not only will ads get more expensive over time, but users will get more and more accustomed to them and ignore them even more than they do today.

How about you? What do *you* think when you see an ad from somebody about something you've never heard of? That's right, you don't think. You ignore. That's the point.

Apply that logic to your business: Why would you send out a Facebook ad trying to convince internet strangers you're an expert *before* you would reach out to people who already know you?

Trying to figure out the best Facebook ad that works right now isn't how you build a business. Even if you're able to "master Facebook advertising" today, things will change tomorrow and you'll be forced to reinvent

---

An exaggeration. It's usually only a few funnels with little to no thought as to how they're going to get anybody funneling through their funnels that they built because, you know, if you build a funnel, they will come. But this ain't Wayne's World, *and no weird naked Indian is going to lead you to Jim Morrison who is going to lead you to the promised land (and when you wake up your football phone finally arrives). Unfortunately, real life doesn't work that way.*

yourself. Back to square one ... "How are you guys getting clients?"

Referrals, recommendations, and mentions hold considerably more weight. I don't see a movie unless at least a few of my friends have already seen it and said it was good. I'd never hire an online trainer I've never heard of no matter how good the sales copy is.

Closer to home for me, I don't expect anybody to enroll in the Online Trainer Academy without getting to know us for a while.

This is how people buy things today.

Paid ads, and any other strategy that asks a client to take a leap to work with you, are tactics, nothing more, nothing less. And tactics are great. I'm not against them. I use them, and they work. But tactics only take out the low-hanging fruit and they should never, ever come first. Advertising on social media is best used to begin a relationship that is then nurtured over time. This requires a back end of content and marketing materials and community that you may or may not yet have in place and, if you don't, takes a lot of time and money to produce.

For these reasons, talking to people comes first. Developing unbelievable relationships, authority, and trust come first.

Build a foundation of people who know, like, and trust you and your selling position shifts from this...

You: Hey client, you should work with me!

Client: Um ... why?

To this...

Client: Hey trainer, how can I work with you?*

The majority of people operate in the first scenario and it contributes to a lot of the frustration I see. Change your sales mindset right now. There's no trickery with sales, no secrets. Sales is the process of figuring out what somebody wants, identifying whether you're properly suited to help, and, if so, positioning yourself and your services in a way that makes the choice easy.

Learning this can take time and practice, but it's imperative for your success.

HOW MANY PEOPLE HAVE YOU SPOKEN TO TODAY?

Make this your daily ritual: Have a conversation with at least five new people every day. It's easy and can lead to so many interesting places.

Listen to Alicia Wagner, an OTA graduate living

---

* *At the Online Trainer Academy, we teach attraction marketing, not push marketing. Our students learn how to put the chess pieces in place to efficiently attract the right kind of people, ready to buy, so that they don't have to beg for attention. It's much nicer this way for everybody. (And yes, we also include a full minicourse of bonus training on Facebook advertising in the Online Trainer Academy, though most of our students never need to use it.)*

in Missouri: "Do not skip the daily ritual. Even if you don't manage it every day, do it as much as you can. This business is about building relationships. At first, I was questioning if it was worth my time. To my surprise, a day later one message I sent turned into a client. I didn't even have to sell her on my services."

When reaching out and building these loose connections, it's not your job to sell. It's your job to be genuine, to show each person you talk to that you care about them and what's happening in their lives, and that you're always happy to help.

The more loose connections you can build with that goal, the more clients will come to you "pre-sold" the way Alicia experienced.

But the time will come when you *will* have to sell

Sure, in an ideal world every single client would come to you completely sold and ready to work, but that's not very realistic. No matter how genuine your message is, no matter how often you're communicating and nurturing the relationships in your network, you're going to find yourself in a position where you need to confidently sell yourself and your services. What will you do?

You'll be ready, because you'll already know two things:

1. The deep-rooted reasons your clients/prospects want to change and live a healthier life (their "why").
2. Exactly how your services help them achieve that goal.

The foundation of that second part is understanding what online training is and how to communicate it highlighting the benefits to the client in addition to the advantages and disadvantages between traditional and online coaching. Many people don't know online training exists, or they do and don't fully grasp the concept. It's your job to make it sound like the greatest-thing-since-sliced-bread breakthrough that it is.

Here's a useful exercise. Below are one-sentence, one-paragraph, and one-page descriptions of what online training is. Master them. Add your own flourishes, or just make up your own. Make 'em yours and be ready when people ask, and feel free to add this to your marketing materials in social media and on your website.

Online training in one sentence:

Option 1: Online training is a new and exciting way for me to offer my clients what they need, when they need it, without the limitations and expenses of the gym, and in a more cost-effective way than in-person training.

Option 2: Online training is a new and exciting way

for me to offer cost-effective body transformation coaching for (insert your type of client here) without the limitations and expenses of the gym.

Option 2 (with example filled in): Online training is a new and exciting way for me to offer more effective, and cost-effective, body transformation coaching for dads who want to get ripped but don't want to deal with the limitations and expenses of the gym.

Option 3: Online training is a new and exciting way to offer health and fitness guidance that can be utilized by anyone from anywhere, offering convenience, responsiveness, flexibility, and affordability.

Option 4: Online training is a location-independent and more affordable way to get the services of a fitness professional, particularly for busy people who value their time. (Credit to Yegor Adamovich)

Online training in one paragraph:

Online training is a new and exciting way to offer life-changing transformation and fitness coaching to clients. It can be utilized by anyone, anywhere, offering convenience, responsiveness, flexibility, and affordability. Best of all, I can empower my clients with more accountability and support than I ever could in person.

Online training in one page (perfect for a website):

Online training is a new and exciting way to offer life-changing transformation and fitness coaching to clients. It can be utilized by anyone, anywhere, offering convenience, responsiveness, flexibility, and affordability. I'm now able to empower my clients with more accountability and support than I ever could in person.

Leveraging the power of the internet and cutting out the overhead costs of the gym means that you get more for your hard-earned dollar. Online platforms and mobile communication tools keep me wired and accessible to my clients even if they're hundreds or thousands of miles away.

Simply put: My online clients get SO much more from me than an in-person clientele ever could.

The best part? The program is your program. No longer limited by rules of the gym, scheduling necessities, and financial obligations to a host of other parties, I can give you precisely what you need, when you need it.

Throw the word "training" out the window. I will be your concierge — giving you what you need, when you need it, no matter how those needs may change over time.

Dealing with objections

Yeah, that's the big wall all salespeople have to climb or slip around or just plain break through: Getting to yes. One of the most basic objections you'll come across will be skepticism of online training itself, but now you have some ammo for that. Other objections will run the gamut, so let's discuss how to handle two of the most common:

1. "It's too expensive/I can't afford it." Remember, if a client understands the value of what you offer, price becomes increasingly irrelevant. If a client doesn't understand the value of what you offer, even the cheapest trainer in the world will be too expensive. Yes, some people can't afford a trainer, but the fact that you're a little cheaper or more expensive than another trainer shouldn't matter. Cost often acts as the fallback if something else is a sticking point. Try to find it. If the client still objects based on price, stay quiet for a few seconds. Often they will talk themselves into the sale. If that doesn't happen, the following conversation flow can be useful if you think the client can afford you but won't commit:

"I totally get it (name). Money can be tight. Is it cool if I tell you a story about another client of mine?"

Potential client says yes.

"Like you, he was committed to training because of (pain points X, Y, and Z) and didn't have clear steps to accomplish his goal of ___. He'd tried a lot before but could never make it work on his own.

"When we met, he was in, but said that his budget didn't allow it. So he waited.

"After a month he was no closer to his goal and he

finally decided to get started. Things moved quickly after that. The added guidance and accountability that he got by training together helped push him, and he reached his goal.

"(Name), you're literally X weeks from hitting your goal on your way to building the body of your dreams, and I want to help you get there. What would it take right now to get you rolling on this program? We made the decision. Let's get you through this. I'm not going to let you down."

2. "I don't have the time." Your clients have taken the time to approach you, or at least listen to you. They wouldn't be there if they weren't interested in training, and they know there must be some time commitment involved. That said, some people are truly more pressed for time than others. Decide if you want to manipulate the prescribed programming to meet their needs. For example, if one client wants to lose fat, you could explain the benefits of "quickie" 25-minute metabolic sessions. You could also suggest a combination of in-gym and at-home workouts. With a little out-of-the-box thinking, you could probably come up with a number of time-saving options.

The best way to introduce an alternate scenario is to say, "You know, you remind me of a client I used to have. His name was __. Can I tell you his story?"

Then tell the story of that client, highlighting a place or two where his story is similar to that of the person you're talking to, and detail how he didn't have time and you altered the program for him. You'll find it's much better to sell through story then by changing the program.

That said, only present these alternatives if you truly believe you can help this client with the adapted program. Otherwise, be honest. Let all clients know that for what they want to achieve, this is the time required. Explain that if they aren't able to put forth that time commitment, they may need to rethink their goals.

Typically, objections are another way your prospect is saying, "I'm not sold on you/this yet." Pinpointing the root of their objection and speaking directly to it is the recipe to overcome.

If your prospect still isn't ready? No problem. Don't rush him. Wish him well, ensure he knows that you're always there to help, and follow up occasionally. That's the funny thing about "no." It often evolves into "yes" over time.

THE TAKEAWAY

While you'll be tempted to use sales tactics on potential clients, true selling is about developing relationships, trust, and your reputation. Good word-of-mouth will do more for your sales than any advertising tactic.

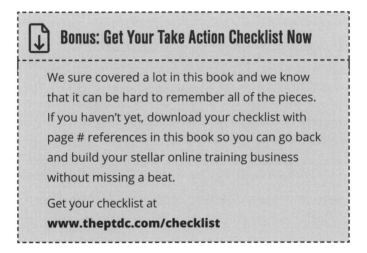

Bonus: Get Your Take Action Checklist Now

We sure covered a lot in this book and we know that it can be hard to remember all of the pieces. If you haven't yet, download your checklist with page # references in this book so you can go back and build your stellar online training business without missing a beat.

Get your checklist at
www.theptdc.com/checklist

AFTERWORD

It's time to take your next step...

...and I'm excited for you.

Every fit pro's business must have a digital component. It's the logical next step in your fulfilling and prosperous career. Having an online training option is better for your clients — allowing you to offer a more flexible service that provides them with precisely what they need, how they need it, in a manner most convenient to them.

For you, it's an opportunity to take back control, win space, and earn your freedom.

As you've seen with all those real-life examples of our students, some fit pros use this newfound freedom to acquire the skills and scale their digital fitness business to six and seven figures.

Others decide that their desire for travel, volunteerism, or family take priority and they're happy with an extra $1,000 to $3,000 per month ($12,000 to $36,000 per year).

Meanwhile, others decide to convert their passion for fitness into a side hustle and enter another industry.

Online training gives you freedom and control. What you do with that freedom is your choice, and that's the point.

This book provided you with the blueprint to get started training online. From setting your foundation to identifying your ideal online client and packaging, pricing, marketing, and selling — you have everything you need to get going.

Still, I know that some fit pros are serious about jump-starting their success and ready to invest even more, knowing that an investment in themselves is the best money they could ever spend. If that's you, then I invite you to enroll in the Online Trainer Academy (OTA).

OTA isn't just the leading certification on the subject, it's also a world-class business development course and mentorship that walks you through the process of creating your ideal online fitness business.

Upon joining us, we'll mail you the textbook, *The Fundamentals of Online Training*, and provide you with every framework, script, worksheet, and legal document you need. You'll also get unlimited lifetime access to our expert mentors through email, live chat, and one-on-one phone calls that you can book whenever, and as often, as you desire.

Not only that, but your enrollment qualifies for our

ironclad 10-year, 1K Extra guarantee.

If you've already decided to join our family by enrolling into the Academy, then I can't wait to work with you. All information and registration can be found at **theptdc.com/ota.** (For your convenience, we also offer a flexible payment plan option.)

Whichever path you choose, I'm excited for your future. Thanks for investing some time with Alex and me by reading this book, and I hope we'll talk soon.

—Coach Jon

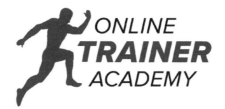

Learn more and enroll today at

www.theptdc.com/ota